Antiarrhythmic Drugs

A practical guide

SECOND EDITION

Richard N. Fogoros, M.D.
Pittsburgh, PA

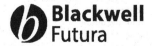

Blackwell
Futura

© 2007 Richard Fogoros
Published by Blackwell Publishing
Blackwell Futura is an imprint of Blackwell Publishing

Blackwell Publishing, Inc., 350 Main Street, Malden, Massachusetts 02148-5020, USA
Blackwell Publishing Ltd, 9600 Garsington Road, Oxford OX4 2DQ, UK
Blackwell Science Asia Pty Ltd, 550 Swanston Street, Carlton, Victoria 3053, Australia

First published 1997
Second edition 2007

1   2007

ISBN: 978-1-4051-6351-4

Library of Congress Cataloging-in-Publication Data

Fogoros, Richard N.
   Antiarrhythmic Drugs : a practical guide / Richard N. Fogoros. – 2nd ed.
      p. ; cm.
   Includes bibliographical references and index.
   ISBN 978-1-4051-6351-4 (alk. paper)
   1. Myocardial depressants.   2. Arrhythmia–Chemotherapy.   I. Title.
   [DNLM: 1. Anti-Arrhythmia Agents.   2. Arrhythmia–drug therapy.
QV 150 F656a 2007]

   RM347.F64 2007
   616.1'28061–dc22

                                                       2007005643

A catalogue record for this title is available from the British Library

Set in Meridien 9.25/12pt by Aptara Inc., New Delhi, India

Commissioning Editor: Gina Almond
Development Editor: Fiona Pattison
Editorial Assistant: Victoria Pitman

For further information on Blackwell Publishing, visit our website:
www.blackwellcardiology.com

Contents

Preface, v

Aknowledgments, viii

Part 1 Basic principles

Chapter 1 Mechanisms of cardiac tachyarrhythmias, 3

Chapter 2 Introduction to antiarrhythmic drugs, 36

Part 2 Clinical features of antiarrhythmic drugs

Chapter 3 Class I antiarrhythmic drugs, 55

Chapter 4 Class II antiarrhythmic drugs; beta-blocking agents, 80

Chapter 5 Class III antiarrhythmic drugs, 86

Chapter 6 Class IV drugs: calcium-blocking agents, 102

Chapter 7 Unclassified antiarrhythmic agents, 107

Chapter 8 Investigational antiarrhythmic drugs, 112

Chapter 9 Common adverse events with antiarrhythmic drugs, 117

Part 3 Antiarrhythmic drugs in the treatment of cardiac arrhythmias

Chapter 10 Basic principles of using antiarrhythmic drugs, 133

Chapter 11 Treatment of supraventricular tachyarrhythmias, 138

Chapter 12 Treatment of ventricular arrhythmias, 151

Chapter 13 Treatment of arrhythmias in pregnancy, 164

Index, 169

Preface

Physicians once found it convenient to think of cardiac arrhythmias as a sort of "itch" of the heart and of antiarrhythmic drugs as a soothing balm that, applied in sufficient quantities, would relieve the itch. During the past several decades, however, pioneering work has revealed many of the complexities of cardiac arrhythmias and of the drugs used to treat them. To the dismay of most reasonable people, the old, convenient viewpoint finally proved utterly false.

Indeed, in the decade since the first edition of this book appeared, the widespread notion that antiarrhythmic drugs are a salve for the irritated heart has been, appropriately, completely reversed. Every clinician worth his or her salt now realizes that antiarrhythmic drugs are among the most toxic substances used in medicine, they are as likely as not to provoke even more dangerous arrhythmias, and, indeed, the use of most of these drugs in most clinical situations has been associated with an increase (and not a decrease) in mortality.

This newfound respect for (if not fear of) antiarrhythmic drugs has been accompanied by the comforting murmurs of an elite army of electrophysiologists, assuring less adept clinicians that, really, there is no reason to worry about these nasty substances anymore. After all (they say), what with implantable defibrillators, radiofrequency ablation, and other emerging technologies (that, by the way, only *we* are qualified to administer), the antiarrhythmic drug as a serious clinical tool has become nearly obsolete.

It is certainly true that the use of antiarrhythmic drugs has been considerably curtailed over the past decade or so and that other emerging treatments have led to significantly improved outcomes for many patients with cardiac arrhythmias. But neither the widely acknowledged shortcomings of these drugs nor the dissemination of new technologies has eliminated the usefulness of antiarrhythmic drugs or obviated the need to apply them, when appropriate, in the treatment of patients with cardiac arrhythmias.

Consider that implantable defibrillators, while in clinical use for over 25 years, are still indicated for only a tiny proportion of patients who are at increased risk of arrhythmic death and are actually implanted in only a small proportion of these. Until these devices are made far cheaper, easier to implant, and more reliable than they are today (changes that would require dramatic—and thus unlikely—alterations in the business models of both the companies that make them and the doctors who implant them), they will never be used in the vast majority of patients who are at risk of arrhythmic death. And consider that ablation techniques to cure atrial fibrillation—the arrhythmia that produces the greatest cumulative morbidity across the population—have failed, despite prolonged and dedicated efforts, to become sufficiently effective or safe for widespread use. And finally, consider that with a deeper understanding of cellular electrophysiology, drug companies are now beginning to "tailor" new compounds that might be more effective and less toxic than those in current use, and that some future generation of antiarrhythmic drugs—possibly even some of the investigational drugs discussed herein—may offer a very attractive alternative to certain expensive or risky technologies.

It remains important, therefore, for any health-care professional caring for patients who are at risk of developing cardiac arrhythmias (and not just the electrophysiologists) to understand something about antiarrhythmic drugs. Accordingly, this book is intended for nonexperts—the practitioners, trainees, and students—who are most often called upon to make decisions regarding actual patients with cardiac arrhythmias. The book attempts to set out a framework for understanding antiarrhythmic drugs: how they work, what they actually do to improve (or worsen) the cardiac rhythm, and the factors one must consider in deciding when and how to use them. Such a framework, it is hoped, will not only serve as a guidepost in making clinical decisions, but will also provide a basis for interpreting new information that comes to light on antiarrhythmic drugs and their place in the treatment of cardiac arrhythmias.

The book is divided into three parts. Part 1 is an introduction to basic principles—the mechanism of cardiac arrhythmias and how antiarrhythmic drugs work. Part 2 discusses the clinically relevant features of the drugs themselves, including emerging investigational drugs that appear to show promise. Part 3 draws on this basic information to explore the treatment of specific cardiac arrhythmias and emphasizes the current roll of antiarrhythmic drugs in managing these arrhythmias.

Throughout this book, basic principles are emphasized. Accordingly, when a choice had to be made between simplicity and complexity, simplicity prevailed in almost every case. The author recognizes that some colleagues may not agree with an approach that risks oversimplification of an inherently complex topic. It is an approach, however, that reflects a deep-seated belief—by keeping the basics simple, the specifics (clinical cases and scientific reports) can be more readily weighed, categorized, absorbed, and implemented.

Acknowledgments

The author thanks Gina Almond, Publisher at Blackwell Publishing, for asking me to consider writing a second edition to this book, and Fiona Pattison, Senior Development Editor at Blackwell, for helping to shepherd me through the process of actually doing so. Their expertise and encouragement is much appreciated. The author also thanks Anne, Emily, and Joe Fogoros for once again overlooking the temporary inattentiveness that always seems to accompany such endeavors.

Part 1

Basic principles

CHAPTER 1

Mechanisms of cardiac tachyarrhythmias

Using antiarrhythmic drugs safely is difficult. Indeed, it is nearly impossible without a firm understanding of the basic mechanisms of cardiac tachyarrhythmias and the basic concepts of how antiarrhythmic drugs work. Part 1 of this book covers these basics. Chapter 1 reviews the normal electrical system of the heart and the mechanisms and clinical features of the major cardiac tachyarrhythmias. Chapter 2 examines the principles of how antiarrhythmic drugs affect arrhythmias.

The electrical system of the heart

On a very fundamental level, the heart is an electrical organ. The electrical signals generated by the heart not only cause muscle contraction (by controlling the flux of calcium ions across the cardiac cell membrane) but also organize the sequence of muscle contraction with each heartbeat, thus optimizing the pumping action of the heart. In addition, and especially pertinent to the subject of this book, the pattern and timing of the cardiac electrical signals determine the heart rhythm. Thus, a well-functioning electrical system is vital for adequate cardiac performance.

Anatomy

The heart's electrical impulse originates in the sinoatrial (SA) node, high in the right atrium near the superior vena cava (Figure 1.1). From the SA node, the impulse spreads radially across both atria. When it reaches the atrioventricular (AV) groove, the impulse encounters the fibrous "skeleton" of the heart, which separates the atria from the ventricles. The fibrous skeleton is electrically inert, and therefore stops the electrical impulse. The only way for the impulse

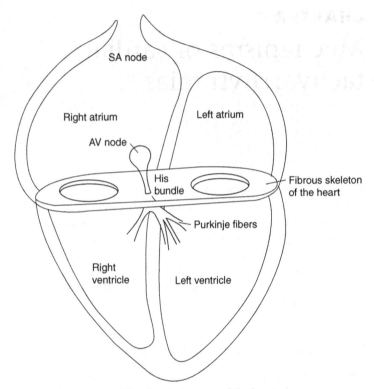

Figure 1.1 Anatomy of the electrical system of the heart.

to cross over to the ventricular side is by means of the specialized AV conducting tissues—the AV node and the His-Purkinje system.

The AV node conducts electricity slowly; when the electrical impulse enters the AV node, its passage is delayed. The delay is reflected in the PR interval on the surface electrocardiogram (ECG). Leaving the AV node, the electrical impulse enters the His bundle, the most proximal part of the rapidly conducting His-Purkinje system. The His bundle penetrates the fibrous skeleton and delivers the impulse to the ventricular side of the AV groove.

Once on the ventricular side, the electrical impulse follows the His-Purkinje system as it divides first into the right and left bundle branches and then into the Purkinje fibers. The Purkinje fibers speed the impulse to the furthermost reaches of the ventricular myocardium. In this way, the electrical impulse is rapidly distributed throughout the ventricles.

The heart's electrical system thus organizes the sequence of my-ocardial contraction with each heartbeat. As the electrical impulse spreads across the atria, the atria contract. The delay provided by the AV node allows complete emptying of the atria before the electrical impulse reaches the ventricles. Once the impulse leaves the AV node, it is distributed rapidly throughout the ventricular muscle by the Purkinje fibers, thus providing brisk and orderly ventricular contraction.

Cardiac action potential

The electrical impulse of the heart is actually the summation of thousands of tiny electrical currents generated by thousands of individual cardiac cells. The electrical activity of an individual cardiac cell is described by the cardiac action potential (Figure 1.2). The action potential is inherently a bit complex and nonintuitive. Fortunately, for our purposes there are only a few things one needs to know about the action potential, and these are reasonably simple to understand.

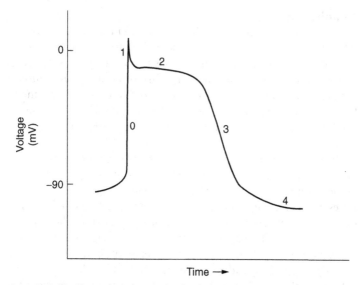

Figure 1.2 Cardiac action potential. Numbers on the curve indicate the five phases of the action potential. Phase 0 corresponds to depolarization. Phases 1–3 correspond to repolarization. Phase 4 corresponds to the resting phase.

The inside of every living cell has a negative electrical charge. The voltage difference across the cell membrane (normally –80 to –90 mV) is called the transmembrane potential and is the result of an accumulation of negatively charged molecules within the cell. The magnitude of the transmembrane potential remains fixed throughout the lives of most living cells.

However, some cells—notably, cardiac cells—are excitable. When excitable cells are stimulated in just the right way, a variety of tiny channels in the cell membrane are induced to open and close in a complex sequence, which allows various electrically charged particles—ions—to pass back and forth across the membrane in an equally complex sequence. The movement of electrical current across the cell membrane occurs in a very stereotypic pattern and leads to a patterned sequence of changes in the transmembrane potential. When the stereotypic changes in voltage are graphed against time, the result is the cardiac action potential.

Although the cardiac action potential is classically divided into five phases (named, somewhat perversely, phases 0 through 4), it is most helpful to consider the action potential in terms of three general phases: depolarization, repolarization, and the resting phase.

Depolarization
The depolarization phase of the action potential, phase 0, occurs when the so-called rapid sodium channels in the cell membrane are stimulated to open, which allows positively charged sodium ions to rush into the cell. The sudden influx of positive ions causes a voltage spike—a rapid, positively directed change in the transmembrane potential. The voltage spike, called *depolarization*, accounts for the heart's electrical impulse; phase 0 is when the "action" of the action potential occurs.

The sodium channels that allow this rapid depolarization are *voltage dependent*; that is, they open when the cell's resting transmembrane potential reaches a certain threshold voltage. The event that raises a cell's transmembrane potential to threshold voltage is most often the depolarization of a nearby cardiac cell. Thus, the depolarization of one cell leads to depolarization of adjacent cells; once a cardiac cell is depolarized, a wave of depolarization (the electrical impulse) tends to spread across the heart, cell by cell.

Further, the speed at which one cell is depolarized (represented by the slope of phase 0) determines how quickly the next cell is stimulated to depolarize, and thus determines the speed at which the electrical impulse is propagated. If something causes the slope of phase 0 to change, the conduction velocity also changes; the faster the depolarization of the cardiac cells, the faster an electrical impulse moves across the heart.

Repolarization

If you fire a Colt 45, you cannot fire it again until you recock it. Similarly, once a cell is depolarized, it cannot be depolarized again until the ionic fluxes that occur during depolarization are reversed. The process of getting the ions back to where they started is called *repolarization*. Repolarization corresponds to phases 1 through 3, and therefore accounts for almost the entire duration of the action potential. Because the cell is refractory to depolarization until after it is repolarized, the time from the end of phase 0 to late in phase 3 is called the *refractory period* of the cell. The duration of the action potential thus determines the refractory period; if one does something to change the duration of the action potential, one also changes the refractory period.

The repolarization of cardiac cells is complex and incompletely understood. Repolarization begins rapidly (phase 1), but the process is almost immediately interrupted by a plateau phase (phase 2), which is unique to cardiac cells (e.g., there is no plateau phase in nerve cells). Phase 2 is mediated by "slow" calcium channels, which allow positively charged calcium ions to enter the cell slowly and thus to interrupt repolarization and prolong the duration of the action potential.

The most important ionic shift that occurs during repolarization is the outward flow of positively charged potassium ions, which has the effect of returning the action potential toward its baseline, negatively polarized state. At least six different potassium "currents" have been identified; they operate at different times during the action potential and are modulated by different factors (including voltage, calcium ions, muscarinic receptors, acetylcholine, and adenosine triphosphate) under different circumstances.

Dumping sodium and calcium ions into a cardiac cell to depolarize it and then draining potassium ions out of the cell to repolarize it may return the transmembrane voltage to baseline levels, but these actions do not return the cell chemistry to the baseline state. Various poorly characterized mechanisms are called on to rectify remaining chemical imbalances (the most important of which is the sodium–potassium pump). Although depolarization seems

fairly straightforward, any attempt to fully understand repolarization quickly leads one into a maze of seemingly conflicting channels,
gates, receptors, and pumps which only a basic electrophysiologist
could love.

Fortunately, the essential features of repolarization are relatively
simple: (1) repolarization returns the cardiac action potential to the
resting transmembrane potential; (2) this process takes time; (3) this
time, roughly corresponding to the width of the action potential,
is the refractory period of cardiac tissue; (4) depolarization mainly
depends on sodium channels, and repolarization mainly depends on
potassium channels.

The resting phase

For most cardiac cells, the resting phase (the period of time between
two action potentials, corresponding to phase 4) is quiescent; there
is no net movement of ions across the cell membrane.

For some cells and in some circumstances, however, the so-called
resting phase is not quiescent. Instead, there is leakage of ions back
and forth across the cell membrane during phase 4 in such a way
as to cause a gradual increase in transmembrane potential (Figure
1.3). When the transmembrane potential reaches the threshold voltage, the appropriate channels are engaged and the cell is depolarized
(since, as noted, the channels mediating depolarization are voltage
dependent). Depolarization, in turn, stimulates nearby cells to depolarize, and the resultant spontaneously generated electrical impulse
is then propagated across the heart. This phase 4 activity, which leads
to spontaneous depolarization, is called automaticity.

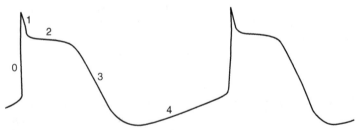

Figure 1.3 Automaticity. In some cardiac cells, leakage of ions across the
cell membrane during phase 4 causes a gradual, positively directed change
in the transmembrane voltage. When the transmembrane voltage becomes
sufficiently positive, the appropriate channels are automatically activated to
generate another action potential. Numbers on the curve indicate phases.

Automaticity is the mechanism by which the normal heart rhythm is generated. Cells in the SA node—the pacemaker of the heart—normally have the fastest phase 4 activity. If for any reason the automaticity of the SA node fails, secondary pacemaker cells (often located in the AV junction) usually take over the pacemaker function of the heart, but they do so at a slower rate because their phase 4 activity is slower.

Localized variations

Two localized differences in the heart's electrical system are important in understanding cardiac arrhythmias: differences in the action potential and differences in autonomic innervation.

Localized differences in the action potential

The cardiac action potential does not have the same shape in every cardiac cell. The action potential shown in Figure 1.2, for instance, represents a typical Purkinje fiber action potential. Figure 1.4 shows the differences in shape among representative action potentials from several key locations of the heart. The action potentials that differ most radically from the Purkinje fiber model are found in the SA node and the AV node. Notice the slow depolarization phases (phase 0) in these action potentials. Slow depolarization occurs

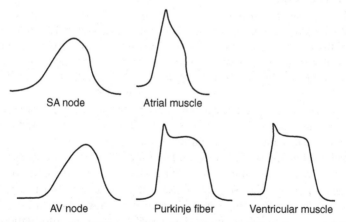

Figure 1.4 Localized differences in cardiac action potential. Action potentials generated in different areas of the heart have different shapes because different electrophysiologic properties (i.e., conduction velocity, refractoriness, and automaticity) are seen in various tissues within the heart.

because the SA nodal and AV nodal tissues lack active, rapid sodium channels and are thought to depend entirely on the slow calcium channel for depolarization. Because the speed of depolarization (the slope of phase 0) determines conduction velocity, the SA and AV nodes conduct electrical impulses slowly.

Localized differences in autonomic innervation

In general, an increase in sympathetic tone causes enhanced automaticity (pacemaker cells fire more rapidly), increased conduction velocity (electrical impulses spread more rapidly), and decreased refractory periods (cells are ready for repeated depolarizations more quickly). Parasympathetic tone has the opposite effect (depressed automaticity, decreased conduction velocity, and increased refractory periods).

Both sympathetic and parasympathetic fibers richly supply the SA and AV nodes. In the remainder of the heart's electrical system, although sympathetic innervation is reasonably abundant, parasympathetic innervation is sparse. Thus, changes in parasympathetic tone have a relatively greater effect on the SA nodal and AV nodal tissues than they do on other tissues of the heart.

Relationship between action potential and surface ECG

The cardiac action potential represents the electrical activity of a single cardiac cell. The surface ECG reflects the electrical activity of the entire heart. Essentially, the ECG represents the summation of all the action potentials of all the cardiac cells. Consequently, the information one gleans from the surface ECG derives from the characteristics of the action potential (Figure 1.5).

In most of the heart, the depolarization phase of a cell is essentially instantaneous (occurring in 1–3 ms), and occurs sequentially from cell to cell. Thus, the instantaneous wave of depolarization can be followed across the heart by studying the ECG. The P wave represents the depolarization front as it traverses the atria; the QRS complex represents the wave of depolarization as it spreads across the ventricles. Because depolarization is relatively instantaneous, the P wave and the QRS complex yield specific directional information. Changes in the spread of the electrical impulse, such as those that occur in bundle branch block or a transmural myocardial infarction, can be readily discerned.

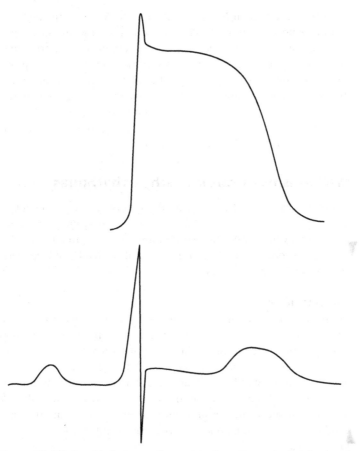

Figure 1.5 Relationship between the ventricular action potential (top) and the surface ECG (bottom). The rapid depolarization phase (phase 0) is reflected by the QRS complex on the ECG. Because phase 0 is almost instantaneous, the QRS complex yields directional information on ventricular depolarization. In contrast, the repolarization portion of the action potential (phases 1–3) has significant duration. Consequently, the portion of the surface ECG that reflects repolarization (the ST segment and the T wave) yields little directional information.

In contrast, the repolarization phase of the action potential is not instantaneous; indeed, repolarization has significant duration, lasting hundreds of times longer than depolarization. Thus, although depolarization occurs from cell to cell sequentially, repolarization of the cells overlaps; all the repolarizations can be thought of as occurring simultaneously. For this reason, the ST segment and the T wave (the portions of the surface ECG that reflect ventricular repolarization) give very little directional information, and abnormalities in the ST segments and T waves are most often (and quite properly) interpreted as being nonspecific. The QT interval represents the time from the beginning of depolarization (the beginning of the QRS complex) to the end of repolarization (the end of the T wave) of the ventricular myocardium, and thus reflects the average action potential duration of ventricular muscle.

Mechanisms of cardiac tachyarrhythmias

Most rapid cardiac arrhythmias are thought to be due to one of two general mechanisms: abnormal automaticity or reentry. In recent years, however, a third general mechanism—the "channelopathy"—has been recognized as the cause of several relatively unusual varieties of cardiac arrhythmias.

Automaticity

As already noted, automaticity is an important feature of the normal electrical system; the pacemaker function of the heart depends upon it. Under some circumstances, however, abnormal automaticity can occur. When an abnormal acceleration of phase 4 activity occurs at some location within the heart, an automatic tachyarrhythmia is the result. Such an automatic focus can arise in the atria, the AV junction, or the ventricles and can lead to automatic atrial tachycardia, automatic junctional tachycardia, or automatic ventricular tachycardia.

Automatic tachyarrhythmias are not particularly common; they probably account for less than 10% of all tachyarrhythmias. Further, automatic tachyarrhythmias are usually recognizable by their characteristics and the clinical settings in which they occur. Consideration of some of the features of sinus tachycardia, which is the only normal variety of automatic tachycardia, may be helpful in this regard. Sinus tachycardia usually occurs as a result of appropriately increased sympathetic tone (e.g., in response to exercise). When sinus tachycardia develops, the heart rate gradually increases from the basic (resting) sinus rate; when sinus tachycardia subsides, the rate likewise decreases gradually.

Similarly, automatic tachyarrhythmias often display "warm-up" and "warm-down" in rate when the arrhythmia begins and ends.

Also, analogous to sinus tachycardia, automatic tachyarrhythmias often have metabolic causes, such as acute cardiac ischemia, hypoxemia, hypokalemia, hypomagnesemia, acid–base disturbances, high sympathetic tone, or the use of sympathomimetic agents. Therefore, automatic arrhythmias are frequently seen in acutely ill patients, usually in the intensive care unit (ICU) setting.

Common examples of automatic tachyarrhythmias are the multifocal atrial tachycardias (MATs) that accompany acute exacerbations of chronic pulmonary disease, many of the atrial and ventricular tachyarrhythmias seen during the induction of and recovery from general anesthesia (probably a result of surges in sympathetic tone), and the ventricular arrhythmias seen during the first minutes to hours of an acute myocardial infarction. (Enhanced automaticity in this situation is thought to be mediated by ischemia.)

Of all tachyarrhythmias, automatic arrhythmias are closest to resembling an "itch" of the heart. The balm of antiarrhythmic drugs is occasionally helpful, but the primary treatment of these arrhythmias should always be directed toward identifying and treating the underlying metabolic cause. In general, these "ICU arrhythmias" resolve once the patient's acute medical problems have been stabilized.

Reentry

The mechanism of reentry accounts for most clinically significant tachyarrhythmias. Recognition of this fact and of the fact that reentrant arrhythmias are amenable to study in the laboratory led to the widespread proliferation of electrophysiology laboratories in the 1980s.

The mechanism of reentry, although less intuitive than the mechanism of automaticity, can still be reduced to a few simple concepts. Reentry cannot occur unless certain underlying conditions exist (Figure 1.6). First, two roughly parallel conducting pathways must be connected proximally and distally by conducting tissue, thus forming a potential electrical circuit. Second, one pathway must have a longer refractory period than the other pathway. Third, the pathway with the shorter refractory period must conduct electrical impulses more slowly than does the opposite pathway.

If all these seemingly implausible conditions are met, reentry can be initiated by introducing an appropriately timed premature impulse to the circuit (Figure 1.7). The premature impulse must enter the circuit early enough that the pathway with the long refractory period is still refractory from the latest depolarization, but late

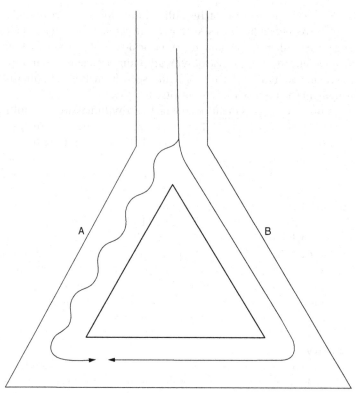

Figure 1.6 Prerequisites for reentry. An anatomic circuit must be present in which two portions of the circuit (pathways A and B) have electrophysiologic properties that differ from one another in a critical way. In this example, pathway A conducts electrical impulses more slowly than pathway B; pathway B has a longer refractory period than pathway A.

enough that the pathway with the shorter refractory period has recovered and is able to conduct the premature impulse. The impulse enters the pathway with the shorter refractory period but is conducted slowly because that pathway has the electrophysiologic property of slow conduction. By the time the impulse reaches the long-refractory-period pathway from below, that pathway has had time to recover and is able to conduct the impulse in the retrograde direction. If the retrograde impulse now reenters the first pathway and is conducted antegradely (as is likely because of the short refractory period of the first pathway), a continuously circulating impulse is established, which rotates around and around the reentrant

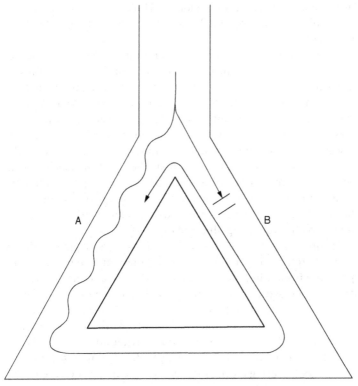

Figure 1.7 Initiation of reentry. If the prerequisites described in Figure 1.6 are present, an appropriately timed, premature electrical impulse can block in pathway A (which has a relatively long refractory period) while conducting down pathway A. Because conduction down pathway A is slow, pathway B has time to recover, allowing the impulse to conduct retrogradely up pathway B. The impulse can then reenter pathway A. A continuously circulating impulse is thus established.

circuit. All that is necessary for the reentrant impulse to usurp the rhythm of the heart is for the impulse to exit from the circuit at some point during each lap and thereby depolarize the remaining myocardium outside the circuit.

Because reentry depends on critical differences in the conduction velocities and refractory periods among the various pathways of the circuit, and because conduction velocities and refractory periods, as we have seen, are determined by the shape of the action potential, the action potentials of the two pathways in any reentrant circuit must be different from one another. Thus, drugs that change the shape of the action potential might be useful in the treatment of reentrant arrhythmias.

Reentrant circuits, while always abnormal, occur with some frequency in the human heart. Some reentrant circuits are present at birth, notably those causing supraventricular tachycardias (e.g., reentry associated with AV bypass tracts and with dual AV nodal tracts). However, reentrant circuits that cause ventricular tachycardias are almost never congenital, but come into existence as cardiac disease develops during life. In the ventricles, reentrant circuits arise in areas in which normal cardiac tissue becomes interspersed with patches of fibrous (scar) tissue, thus forming potential anatomic circuits. Thus, ventricular reentrant circuits usually occur only when fibrosis develops in the ventricles, such as after a myocardial infarction or with cardiomyopathic diseases.

Theoretically, if all anatomic and electrophysiologic criteria for reentry are present, any impulse that enters the circuit at the appropriate instant in time induces a reentrant tachycardia. The time from the end of the refractory period of the shorter-refractory-period pathway to the end of the refractory period of the pathway with a longer refractory time, during which reentry can be induced, is called the *tachycardia zone*. Treating reentrant arrhythmias often involves trying to narrow or abolish the tachycardia zone with antiarrhythmic drugs (by using a drug that, one hopes, might increase the refractory period of the shorter-refractory-period pathway, or decrease the refractory period of the longer-refractory-period pathway).

Because reentrant arrhythmias can be reproducibly induced (and terminated) by appropriately timed impulses, these arrhythmias are ideal for study in the electrophysiology laboratory. In many instances (very commonly with supraventricular arrhythmias, but only occasionally with ventricular arrhythmias), the pathways involved in the reentrant circuit can be precisely mapped, the effect of various therapies can be assessed, and critical portions of the circuit can even be ablated through the electrode catheter.

The channelopathies

In recent years, some varieties of tachyarrhythmias have been attributed to genetic abnormalities in the channels that mediate ionic fluxes across the cardiac cell membrane. Such "channelopathies"—abnormally functioning channels due to inheritable mutations—can affect any electrically active cell and are not limited to the heart. For instance, some varieties of migraine, epilepsy, periodic paralysis, and muscle disorders are apparently due to channelopathies.

While several distinctive cardiac arrhythmias are now thought to be caused by channelopathies, the most clinically relevant and the most common channelopathic arrhythmias are those related to triggered activity.

Triggered activity

Triggered activity is caused by abnormal fluxes of positive ions into cardiac cells. These ionic fluxes produce an abnormal "bump" in the action potential during late phase 3 or early phase 4 (Figure 1.8). The bump is called an afterdepolarization. In most if not all cases, afterdepolarizations are thought to be due to inherited abnormalities in the channels that control the movement of calcium ions across the cell membrane. If the afterdepolarizations are of sufficient amplitude, they can trigger the rapid sodium channels (which, as noted, are voltage dependent), and thus cause another action potential to be generated.

Digitalis-toxic arrhythmias, torsades de pointes, and some of the rare ventricular tachycardias that respond to calcium-blocking agents have all been advanced as arrhythmias that are most likely caused by triggered activity.

Clinical features of the major tachyarrhythmias

Before considering how antiarrhythmic drugs work, it will be helpful to review the salient clinical features of the major cardiac tachyarrhythmias.

Supraventricular tachyarrhythmias

Table 1.1 classifies the supraventricular tachyarrhythmias according to mechanism.

Automatic supraventricular tachyarrhythmias

Automatic supraventricular arrhythmias are seen almost exclusively in acutely ill patients, most of whom have one of the following conditions: myocardial ischemia, acute exacerbations of chronic lung disease, acute alcohol toxicity, or major electrolyte disturbances. Any of these disorders can produce ectopic automatic foci in the atrial myocardium.

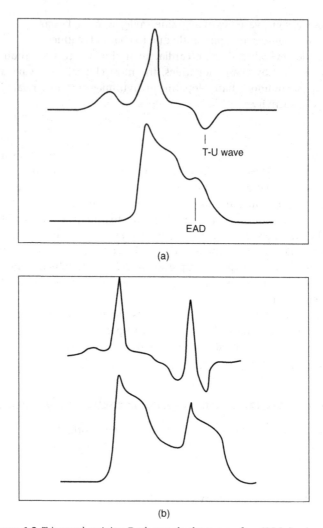

Figure 1.8 Triggered activity. Both panels show a surface ECG (top) and a simultaneous ventricular action potential (bottom). (a) Phase 3 of the action potential is interrupted by a "bump"—an EAD. The EAD is reflected on the surface ECG by a prolonged and distorted T wave (T-U wave). (b) The EAD is of sufficient amplitude to engage the rapid sodium channel and generate another action potential. The resultant premature complex is seen on surface ECG. Note that just as the premature action potential is coincident with the EAD (since it is generated by the EAD), the premature ventricular complex is also coincident with the T-U wave of the previous complex.

Table 1.1 Classification of supraventricular tachyarrhythmias

Automatic arrhythmias
   Some atrial tachycardias associated with acute medical conditions
   Some multifocal atrial tachycardias

Reentrant arrhythmias
   SA nodal reentrant tachycardia
   Intra-atrial reentrant tachycardia
   Atrial flutter and atrial fibrillation
   AV nodal reentrant tachycardia
   Macroreentrant (bypass-mediated) reentrant tachycardia

Triggered arrhythmias (probable mechanism)
   Digitalis-toxic atrial tachycardia
   Some multifocal atrial tachycardias

SA, sinoatrial; AV, atrioventricular.

Clinically, the heart rate with automatic atrial tachycardias is usually less than 200 beats/min. Like all automatic rhythms, the onset and offset are usually relatively gradual; that is, they often display warm-up, in which the heart rate accelerates over several cardiac cycles. Each QRS complex is preceded by a discrete P wave, whose shape generally differs from the normal sinus P wave, depending on the location of the automatic focus within the atrium. Likewise, the PR interval is often shorter than it is during sinus rhythm, since the ectopic focus may be relatively close to the AV node. Because automatic atrial tachycardias arise in and are localized to the atrial myocardium (and thus the arrhythmia itself is not dependent on the AV node), if AV block is produced, atrial arrhythmia itself is unaffected.

MAT (Figure 1.9) is the most common form of automatic atrial tachycardia. It is characterized by multiple (usually at least three) P-wave morphologies and irregular PR intervals. MAT is thought to be caused by the presence of several automatic foci within the atria, firing at different rates. The arrhythmia is usually associated with exacerbation of chronic lung disease, especially in patients receiving theophylline.

Pharmacologic therapy is usually not very helpful in treating automatic atrial tachycardia, though drugs that affect the AV node can

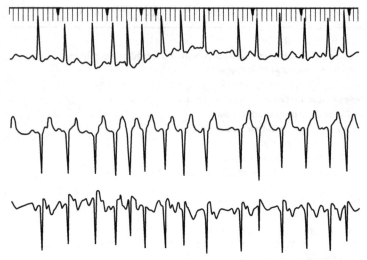

Figure 1.9 MAT is an irregular atrial tachyarrhythmia that superficially resembles atrial fibrillation. However, in MAT (in contrast to atrial fibrillation), each QRS complex is preceded by a discrete P wave. Further, at least three distinct P-wave morphologies are present, which reflects the multifocal origin of atrial activity in this arrhythmia.

sometimes slow the ventricular rate by creating second-degree block. The basic strategy for treating automatic atrial arrhythmias is to aggressively treat the underlying illness.

Reentrant supraventricular tachyarrhythmias

In general, patients have reentrant supraventricular tachyarrhythmias because they are born with abnormal electrical pathways that create potential reentrant circuits. Accordingly (in contrast to patients with automatic supraventricular arrhythmias), these patients most often initially experience symptoms when they are young and healthy. Most supraventricular tachyarrhythmias seen in otherwise healthy patients are caused by the mechanism of reentry.

The five general categories of reentrant supraventricular arrhythmias are listed in Table 1.1. Many clinicians lump these arrhythmias together (except for atrial fibrillation and atrial flutter, which generally are easily distinguishable) as paroxysmal atrial tachycardia (PAT). In most instances, an astute clinician can tell which specific category of PAT he or she is dealing with (and therefore can institute appropriate therapy) merely by carefully examining a 12-lead ECG of the arrhythmia.

AV nodal reentrant tachycardia

AV nodal reentrant tachycardia is the most common type of PAT, accounting for nearly 60% of regular supraventricular tachyarrhythmias. In AV nodal reentry, the reentrant circuit can be visualized as being enclosed entirely within an AV node that is functionally divided into two separate pathways (Figure 1.10). The dual pathways form the reentrant circuit responsible for the arrhythmia. Because

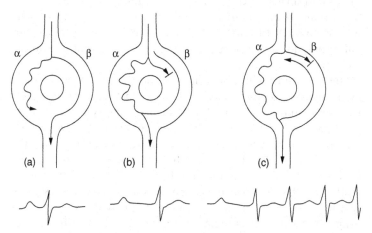

Figure 1.10 AV nodal reentrant tachycardia. (a) In patients with AV nodal reentry, the AV node is functionally divided into two separate pathways (alpha (α) and beta (β) pathways). Similar to the example shown in Figures 1.6 and 1.7, the alpha pathway conducts more slowly than the beta pathway, and the beta pathway has a longer refractory period than the alpha pathway. Since the beta pathway conducts more rapidly than does the alpha pathway, a normal atrial impulse reaches the ventricles via the beta pathway. (b) A premature atrial impulse can find the beta pathway still refractory at a time when the alpha pathway is not refractory. Because conduction down the alpha pathway is slow, the resultant PR interval is prolonged. (c) If conditions are right, a premature impulse can block in the beta pathway and conduct down the alpha pathway (as in (b)), then travel retrograde up the beta pathway and reenter the alpha pathway in the antegrade direction. AV nodal reentrant tachycardia results when such a circuitous impulse is established within the AV node.

the reentrant circuit is within the AV node, the pharmacologic treatment of AV nodal reentry usually involves giving drugs that act upon the AV node.

Bypass-tract-mediated macroreentrant tachycardia

Tachycardia mediated by AV bypass tracts (also called accessory pathways) is the next most common type of reentrant supraventricular tachycardia and accounts for approximately 30% of arrhythmias presenting as PAT. Most patients with such bypass tracts do not have overt Wolff-Parkinson–White syndrome, however. Instead, they have *concealed* bypass tracts, that is, bypass tracts that are incapable of conducting in the antegrade direction (from the atrium to the ventricles), and therefore never display delta waves. Concealed bypass tracts are able to conduct electrical impulses only in the retrograde direction (from the ventricles to the atrium).

The reentrant circuit responsible for these tachycardias is formed by the bypass tract (which almost always constitutes the retrograde pathway), and the normal AV nodal conducting system (the antegrade pathway), connected by the atrial and ventricular myocardium (Figure 1.11). Because the reentrant circuit is large (involving the AV node, the His-Purkinje system, the ventricular myocardium, the bypass tract, and the atrial myocardium), it is termed a *macroreentrant circuit*. Also, because the circuit consists of several types of tissue, it can be attacked on many levels by many different kinds of drugs—drugs that affect the AV node, the bypass tract, the ventricular myocardium, or the atrial myocardium.

Intra-atrial reentry

Intra-atrial reentry accounts for only a small percentage of arrhythmias presenting as PAT. The reentrant circuit in intra-atrial reentry resides entirely within the atrial myocardium and does not involve the AV conducting system (Figure 1.12). Intra-atrial reentry resembles automatic atrial tachycardia because discrete (most often atypical) P waves precede each QRS complex, and AV block can occur without affecting the arrhythmia itself. Intra-atrial reentry differs from automatic tachycardia because of its sudden onset and termination, and, like all reentrant arrhythmias, it can be induced by pacing. Intra-atrial reentry is affected only by drugs that affect the atrial myocardium.

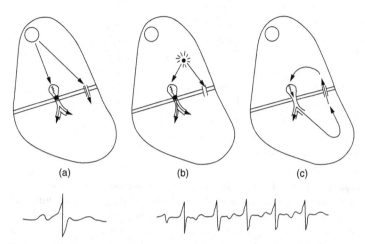

Figure 1.11 Bypass-tract-mediated macroreentrant tachycardia. (a) Because a bypass tract is present, a normal sinus beat is transmitted to the ventricles via two separate pathways. Because the ventricle is partially preexcited (i.e., some ventricular myocardium is depolarized early via the bypass tract), the QRS complex displays a delta wave. A bypass tract usually has a longer refractory period than the normal conducting system, and the normal conducting system includes the slow-conducting AV node and conducts electrical impulses more slowly than the bypass tract. Thus, the substrate for reentry is present. (b) A premature atrial complex occurs during the refractory period of the bypass tract and is therefore conducted solely via the normal conducting system. The resultant QRS complex displays no delta wave. (c) Because conduction via the normal conducting system is relatively slow, the bypass tract may no longer be refractory by the time the impulse reaches the ventricles. Thus, the bypass tract may be able to conduct the impulse retrogradely back to the atrium. If so, a reentrant impulse may be established, which travels antegradely down the normal conducting system and retrogradely up the bypass tract. The result is a large (macro) reentrant circuit.

Atrial flutter and atrial fibrillation

Atrial flutter and atrial fibrillation are special forms of intra-atrial reentrant tachycardias and are generally distinguishable quite readily from other kinds of atrial tachyarrhythmias (commonly labeled PAT) by reviewing a 12-lead ECG.

In atrial flutter, the atrial activity is regular, in excess of 220 beats/min, and usually displays a typical sawtooth pattern (Figure 1.13). Atrial flutter is almost always accompanied by AV block, most often in a 2:1 pattern.

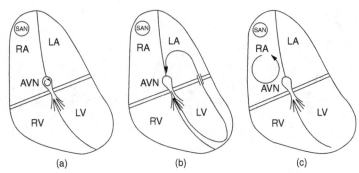

(a)   (b)   (c)

Figure 1.12 The components of the reentrant circuit determine which antiarrhythmic drugs are likely to be effective in treating supraventricular
tachycardia. Both AV nodal reentry (a) and macroreentry (b) include the
AV node within the reentrant circuit. Therefore, drugs that affect the AV
node affect the reentrant circuit itself and may be useful in terminating
or preventing the arrhythmia. In contrast, in intra-atrial reentry (c), the
reentrant circuit does not include the AV node. Drugs that affect the AV
node generally do not affect intra-atrial reentry itself, although they may
be effective in slowing the ventricular response during the arrhythmia.
Atrial fibrillation, atrial flutter, and automatic atrial tachycardia are similar to intra-atrial reentry in that the AV node is not required for initiating or sustaining these arrhythmias. AVN, atrioventricular node; LA, left
atrium; LV, left ventricle; RA, right atrium; RV, right ventricle; SAN, sinoatrial
node.

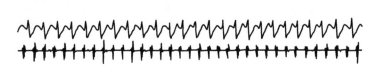

Figure 1.13 Atrial flutter. A surface ECG (top) and an intracardiac electro-
gram that directly records intra-atrial electrical activity (bottom) are shown.
Note the two atrial impulses (seen on the intracardiac electrogram) for every
QRS complex; AV block occurs in a typical 2:1 pattern.

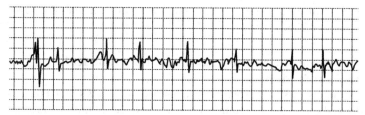

Figure 1.14 Atrial fibrillation. Note the randomly irregular ventricular response and the absence of discrete P waves.

In atrial fibrillation, the atrial activity is continuous and chaotic, and discrete P waves cannot be distinguished (Figure 1.14). The ventricular response is completely irregular, reflecting the chaotic nature of the atrial activity.

Since atrial fibrillation and atrial flutter are intra-atrial arrhythmias, AV block (which occurs in almost every case) does not affect the arrhythmia itself. Drug therapy is usually aimed at converting the arrhythmia by use of drugs that affect the atrial myocardium or at controlling the ventricular response with drugs that affect AV conduction.

SA nodal reentry

SA nodal reentry is a relatively uncommon arrhythmia in which the reentrant circuit is thought to be enclosed entirely within the SA node (i.e., dual SA nodal pathways are thought to exist, similar to those seen in AV nodal reentry). Discrete P waves identical to sinus P waves precede each QRS complex. SA nodal reentry is distinguishable from normal sinus tachycardia (which is automatic in mechanism) by its sudden onset and offset, and by the fact that it is inducible with pacing. It is affected by drugs that affect the SA and AV nodes.

Triggered supraventricular tachyarrhythmias

The only supraventricular tachycardia commonly attributed to triggered activity is that seen with digitalis toxicity. Digitalis toxicity can produce delayed afterdepolarizations (DADs; see Figure 1.16a) that can lead to atrial tachycardias. Clinically, since digitalis toxicity also produces AV block, digitalis-toxic arrhythmias often manifest as atrial tachycardia with block. In fact, the presence of atrial tachycardia with block should always make one consider the possibility of digitalis toxicity.

Electrocardiographic patterns of supraventricular tachyarrhythmias

Often it is possible to specifically diagnose a patient's supraventricular arrhythmia by examining a 12-lead ECG. Atrial flutter and atrial fibrillation can usually be distinguished by simple inspection. In the supraventricular tachycardias commonly labeled as PAT (i.e., regular, narrow-complex tachycardias), both the relationship of the P waves to the QRS complexes and the morphology of the P waves during the tachycardia can be very helpful. Figure 1.15 shows the essential electrocardiographic characteristics of the four types of PAT.

Ventricular tachyarrhythmias

Table 1.2 classifies the ventricular tachyarrhythmias according to mechanism.

Automatic ventricular tachyarrhythmias

Abnormal automaticity accounts for a relatively small proportion of ventricular tachyarrhythmias. As is the case with automatic atrial arrhythmias, automatic ventricular arrhythmias are usually associated with acute medical conditions, such as myocardial ischemia, acid–base disturbances, electrolyte abnormalities, and high adrenergic tone. Automatic ventricular arrhythmias are most often seen in patients with acute myocardial ischemia or infarction, or some other acute medical illness. Most arrhythmias occurring within the first few hours of an acute myocardial infarction are thought to be automatic. Once the ischemic tissue dies or stabilizes, however, the substrate for automaticity is no longer present.

In general, the treatment of automatic ventricular arrhythmias consists of treating the underlying illness. Antiarrhythmic drugs are occasionally beneficial.

Reentrant ventricular tachyarrhythmias

Most ventricular arrhythmias are reentrant in mechanism. While the conditions producing automatic ventricular arrhythmias are usually temporary in nature (e.g., cardiac ischemia), the substrate necessary for producing reentrant ventricular arrhythmias, once present, tends to be permanent.

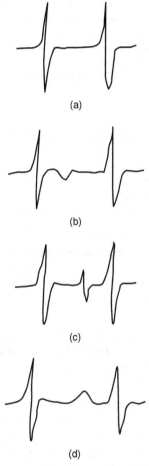

(a)

(b)

(c)

(d)

Figure 1.15 Typical P-wave relationships in four kinds of PAT. Surface ECG lead II is depicted. (a) In AV nodal reentrant tachycardia, the P wave is usually buried within the QRS complex and is most often not discernible even with careful study of all 12-lead ECG. (b) In bypass-tract-mediated macroreentrant tachycardia, the inferior ECG leads usually show a negative P wave. (It has a superior axis because the atria are activated in the retrograde direction.) Also, the P wave is usually closer to the preceding QRS complex than to the following QRS complex. (c) In intra-atrial reentry, discrete P waves almost always are seen before each QRS complex. Because the intra-atrial reentrant circuit can be located anywhere within the atria, the P-wave morphology can have any configuration. The PR interval is usually normal or short. (d) In SA nodal reentry, P waves and the PR interval appear normal.

Table 1.2 Classification of ventricular tachyarrhythmias

Automatic arrhythmias
  Some ventricular tachycardias associated with acute medical conditions
  Acute myocardial infarction or ischemia
  Electrolyte and acid–base disturbances or hypoxia
  High sympathetic tone

Reentrant arrhythmias
  Ventricular tachycardia and fibrillation associated with some chronic heart
    diseases
  Previous myocardial infarction
  Dilated cardiomyopathy
  Hypertrophic cardiomyopathy
  Channelopathies

Triggered arrhythmias (probable mechanism)
  Pause-dependent torsades de pointes (EADs) associated with drugs that
    prolong QT interval
  Catechol-dependent torsades de pointes (DADs) associated with digitalis
    toxicity or idiopathy

Brugada syndrome and SUNDS

EADs, early afterdepolarizations; DADs, delayed afterdepolarizations; SUNDS, sudden unexpected nocturnal death syndrome.

Reentrant circuits within the ventricular myocardium usually arise after scar tissue develops, a condition most commonly seen in patients who have myocardial infarctions or cardiomyopathy. Once the scar tissue gives rise to a reentrant circuit, the circuit persists, and the potential for a ventricular arrhythmia always exists. Thus, the "late" sudden deaths that occur after a myocardial infarction (i.e., from about 12 h to several years after the acute event) are usually a result of reentrant arrhythmias. Reentrant ventricular arrhythmias are seen only rarely in individuals who have normal ventricles.

Most antiarrhythmic drugs affect the ventricular myocardium and, accordingly, most are used to treat ventricular tachyarrhythmias.

Channelopathic ventricular tachyarrhythmias
Channelopathies probably account for several distinctive types of ventricular tachyarrhythmias, at least two of which have now been

well characterized. These are the ventricular arrhythmias due to triggered activity and Brugada syndrome.

Triggered activity in the ventricles

Because ventricular tachyarrhythmias due to triggered activity are reasonably common, and because the management of triggered ventricular arrhythmias is very different from the management of more typical ventricular arrhythmias, it is important to recognize their characteristics. Two fairly distinct clinical syndromes are caused by ventricular triggered activity: catechol-dependent arrhythmias and pause-dependent arrhythmias. In each syndrome, the resultant ventricular arrhythmias are similar. They are the classically polymorphic ventricular tachyarrhythmias generally referred to as *torsades de pointes*.

Catechol-dependent triggered arrhythmias. Catechol-dependent triggered arrhythmias are caused by DADs, which occur during phase 4 of the action potential (Figure 1.16a). DADs are seen in susceptible patients in the setting of digitalis intoxication and cardiac ischemia. They are also seen in certain patients who have a congenital form of QT prolongation associated with what is thought to be an imbalance in the sympathetic innervation of the heart, with predominant input coming from the left stellate ganglia—stimulation of which can reproduce DADs.

The ventricular arrhythmias caused by DADs typically are polymorphic, and are seen in conditions of high sympathetic tone. Patients with catechol-dependent triggered activity therefore experience arrhythmias (often manifested by syncope or cardiac arrest) in times of severe emotional stress or during exercise. Often they have normal ECGs at rest but will develop QT abnormalities during exercise. The onset of the arrhythmia is not associated with a pause.

Left stellate sympathectomy has eliminated arrhythmias in some of these patients. Medical treatment has generally consisted of beta blockers and calcium-channel blockers (consistent with the fact that DADs are thought to be mediated by abnormalities in the calcium channels). Many of these patients, however, end up receiving implantable defibrillators.

Pause-dependent triggered arrhythmias. Pause-dependent triggered arrhythmias are caused by afterdepolarizations that occur during

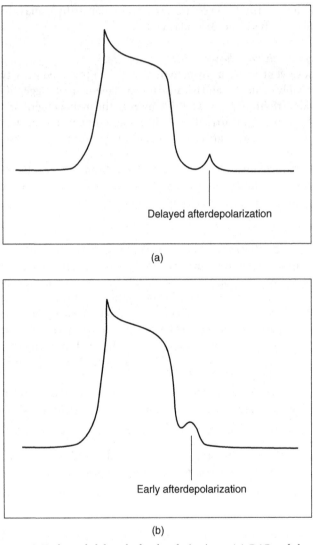

Delayed afterdepolarization

(a)

Early afterdepolarization

(b)

Figure 1.16 Early and delayed afterdepolarizations. (a) DADs of the type thought to be responsible for catechol-dependent triggered arrhythmias. The DAD occurs during phase 4 of the action potential. (b) EAD of the type thought to be responsible for pause-dependent triggered arrhythmias. The EAD occurs during phase 3 of the action potential.

phase 3 of the action potential; hence, they are called early after-depolarizations (EADs; see Figure 1.16b). If the EAD reaches the threshold potential of the cardiac cell, another action potential is generated and an arrhythmia occurs. EADs are generally seen only under circumstances that prolong the duration of the action potential, such as electrolyte abnormalities (hypokalemia and hypomagnesemia), and with the use of certain drugs that cause widening of the action potential, predominantly antiarrhythmic drugs (Table 1.3).

Table 1.3 Drugs that can cause torsades de pointes

Class I and Class III antiarrhythmic drugs
  Quinidine
  Procainamide
  Disopyramide
  Propafenone
  Sotalol
  Amiodarone
  Bretylium
  Ibutilide

Tricyclic and tetracyclic antidepressants
  Amitriptyline
  Imipramine
  Doxepin
  Maprotiline

Phenothiazines
  Thioridazine
  Chlorpromazine

Antibiotics
  Erythromycin
  Trimethoprim-sulfamethoxazole

Others
  Bepridil
  Lidoflazine
  Probucol
  Haloperidol
  Chloral hydrate

It appears that some finite subset of the apparently normal population is susceptible to developing EADs. These patients, from available evidence, have one of several channelopathies that become clinically manifest only when their action potential durations are increased by drugs or electrolyte abnormalities.

The ventricular arrhythmias associated with EADs are typically polymorphic, and most often occur repeatedly and in short bursts, although prolonged arrhythmic episodes, leading to syncope or sudden death, can occur. The repolarization abnormalities responsible for these arrhythmias (i.e., the afterdepolarizations) are reflected on the surface ECG, where the T-wave configuration is often distorted and a U wave is present. The U wave is the ECG manifestation of the EAD itself. The T-U abnormalities tend to be dynamic; that is, they wax and wane from beat to beat, mainly depending on beat-to-beat variations in heart rate. The slower the heart rate, the more exaggerated the T-U abnormality; hence, this condition is said to be pause dependent. Once a burst of ventricular tachycardia is generated (triggered by an EAD that is of sufficient amplitude to reach the threshold potential), it tends to be repeated in a pattern of "ventricular tachycardia bigeminy." An example is shown in Figure 1.17. In this figure, each burst of polymorphic ventricular tachycardia causes a compensatory pause, and the pause causes the ensuing normal beat to be associated with pronounced U-wave abnormalities (i.e., a large EAD). The large EAD, in turn, produces another burst of tachycardia. Pause-dependent triggered activity should be strongly suspected whenever this ECG pattern is seen, especially in the setting of overt QT prolongation or in the setting of conditions that predispose to QT prolongation.

The acute treatment of pause-dependent triggered activity consists of attempting to reduce the duration of the action potential, to eliminate the pauses, or both. Drugs that prolong the QT interval should be immediately discontinued and avoided. Electrolyte abnormalities should be corrected quickly. Intravenous magnesium often ameliorates the arrhythmias even when serum magnesium levels are in the normal range. The mainstay of emergent treatment of the arrhythmias, however, is to eliminate the pauses that trigger the arrhythmias—that is, to increase the heart rate. This is most often accomplished by pacing the atrium or the ventricles (usually, at rates of 100–120 beats/min) or, occasionally, by using an isoproterenol infusion.

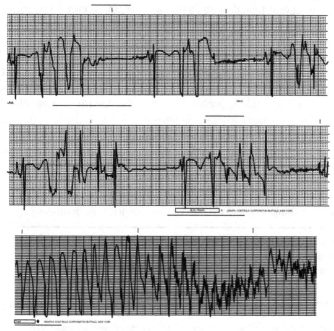

Figure 1.17 Pause-dependent triggered arrhythmias. The figure depicts rhythm strips from a patient who developed torsades de pointes after receiving a Class IA antiarrhythmic agent. The top two strips show the typical pattern—each burst of polymorphic ventricular tachycardia is followed by a compensatory pause; the pause, in turn, causes the ensuing sinus beat to be followed by another burst of ventricular tachycardia. The bottom strip shows the sustained polymorphic ventricular tachycardia that followed after several minutes of ventricular tachycardia bigeminy. Note the broad T-U wave that follows each sinus beat in the top two strips. The T-U wave is thought to reflect the pause-dependent EADs that are probably responsible for the arrhythmia.

Once the underlying cause for the EADs has been reversed, chronic treatment focuses on avoiding conditions that prolong action potential duration.

Brugada syndrome
Brugada syndrome is characterized by ventricular tachyarrhythmias (often causing syncope or cardiac arrest, and often occurring during sleep) in the setting of an underlying characteristic ECG pattern

consisting of unusual, nonishchemic ST-segment elevations in leads V1–V3 and "pseudo" right bundle branch block. Brugada syndrome is usually seen in males and is probably the same disorder as the sudden unexpected nocturnal death syndrome seen in Asian males. Patients with Brugada syndrome have genetic abnormalities in the rapid sodium channel. Several varieties of sodium channelopathies have been identified, probably accounting for the several clinical varieties seen with Brugada syndrome. For instance, in some patients, the characteristic ECG changes are not seen unless a Class I antiarrhythmic drug (i.e., a drug that operates on the sodium channel) is administered. The implantable defibrillator is the mainstay of therapy for patients with Brugada syndrome.

Table 1.4 Clinical features of uncommon ventricular tachycardias

---

Idiopathic left ventricular tachycardia
  Younger patients, no structural heart disease
  Inducible VT with RBBB, superior axis morphology
  Responds to beta blockers and calcium-channel blockers
  Both reentry and triggered activity have been postulated as mechanisms

Right ventricular outflow tract tachycardia (repetitive monomorphic VT)
  Younger patients, no structural heart disease
  VT originates in RV outflow tract; has LBBB, inferior axis morphology; often not
    inducible during EP testing
  Responds to beta blockers, calcium blockers, and transcatheter RF ablation
  Postulated to be due to automaticity or triggered automaticity

Ventricular tachycardia associated with right ventricular dysplasia
  Younger patients with RV dysplasia (portions of RV replaced by fibrous tissue)
  LBBB ventricular tachycardia; almost always inducible during EP testing
  Treatment similar to treatment of reentrant VT in setting of coronary artery
    disease

Bundle branch reentry
  Patients with dilated cardiomyopathy and intraventricular conduction
    abnormality
  Rapid VT with LBBB morphology; reentrant circuit uses RBB in downward
    direction and LBB in upward direction
  Can be cured by RF ablation of RBB

EP, electrophysiologic; LBB, left bundle branch; LBBB, left bundle branch block; RBB, right bundle branch; RBBB, right bundle branch block; RV, right ventricle; VT, ventricular tachycardia.

Miscellaneous ventricular arrhythmias

Several clinical syndromes have been described involving unusual ventricular arrhythmias that do not fit clearly into any of these categories. Nomenclature for these arrhythmias is unsettled in the literature, reflecting the lack of understanding of their mechanisms. Table 1.4 lists the salient features of relatively uncommon ventricular arrhythmias. It is likely that at least some of these will eventually prove to be due to channelopathies. They are discussed in more detail in Chapter 12.

CHAPTER 2

Introduction to antiarrhythmic drugs

All cardiac tachyarrhythmias—whether caused by abnormal auto-maticity, reentry, or channelopathies—are mediated by localized or generalized changes in the cardiac action potential. Thus, it should not be surprising that drugs that alter the action potential might have important effects on cardiac arrhythmias.

How antiarrhythmic drugs work

Thinking of an antiarrhythmic drug as a soothing balm that sup-presses an "irritation of the heart" is more than merely naive; it is dangerous. If this is how one imagines antiarrhythmic drugs to work, then when an arrhythmia fails to respond to a chosen drug, the natural response is to either increase the dosage of the drug or, worse, add additional drugs (in a futile attempt to sufficiently soothe the irritation).

Effect on cardiac action potential
What antiarrhythmic drugs actually do—the characteristic that makes them "antiarrhythmic"—is to change the shape of the car-diac action potential. Antiarrhythmic drugs do this, in general, by altering the channels that control the flow of ions across the cardiac cell membrane.

For example, Class I antiarrhythmic drugs inhibit the rapid sodium channel. As shown in Figure 2.1, the rapid sodium channel is con-trolled by two gates called the m gate and the h gate. In the resting state, the m gate is open and the h gate is closed. When an appro-priate stimulus occurs, the m gate opens, which allows positively charged sodium ions to pour into the cell very rapidly, thus causing the cell to depolarize (phase 0 of the action potential). After a few milliseconds, the h gate closes and sodium stops flowing; phase 0 ends.

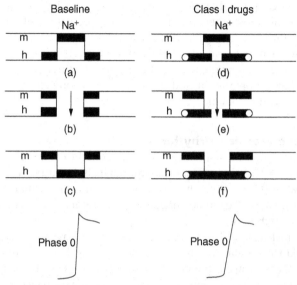

Figure 2.1 The effect of Class I antiarrhythmic drugs on the rapid sodium channel. The sodium channel (Na^+) is controlled by two gates: the m gate and the h gate. Panels (a) through (c) display the function of the two controlling gates in the baseline (drug-free) state. (a) The resting state; the m gate is closed and the h gate is open. (b) The cell is stimulated, causing the m gate to open, which allows positively charged sodium ions to rapidly enter the cell (arrow). (c) The h gate shuts and sodium transport stops (i.e., phase 0 ends). Panels (d) and (e) display the effect of adding a Class I antiarrhythmic drug (open circles). (d) Class I drug binding to the h gate makes the h gate behave as if it is partially closed. (e) The cell is stimulated; the m gate still opens normally, but the channel through which sodium ions enter the cell is narrower, and sodium transport is slower. Consequently, reaching the end of phase 0 takes longer; the slope of phase 0 and the conduction velocity are decreased.

Class I antiarrhythmic drugs work by binding to the h gate, making it behave as if it is partially closed. When the m gate opens, the opening through which sodium enters the cell is functionally much narrower; thus, it takes longer to depolarize the cell (i.e., the slope of phase 0 is decreased). Because the speed of depolarization determines how quickly adjacent cells depolarize (and therefore affects the speed of conduction of the electrical impulse), Class I drugs decrease the conduction velocity of cardiac tissue.

Although not all their precise sites of action have been completely worked out, most other antiarrhythmic drugs operate similarly; they bind to the channels and gates that control the flux of ions across the cardiac cell membrane. In so doing, these drugs change the shape of the cardiac action potential, and thus change the three basic electrophysiologic properties of cardiac tissue: conduction velocity, refractoriness, and automaticity.

Effect on cardiac arrhythmias

Tachyarrhythmias are mediated by changes in the cardiac action potential, whether the mechanism is automaticity, reentry, or a channelopathy. It is not difficult to imagine, then, how drugs that change the shape of the action potential might be useful in treating cardiac tachyarrhythmias.

In practice, the drugs commonly referred to as antiarrhythmic are relatively ineffective in treating automatic arrhythmias or channelopathies. Instead, the potential benefit of these drugs is almost exclusive to the treatment of reentrant arrhythmias, which account for most cardiac arrhythmias. Nonetheless, drugs that change the shape of the action potential can potentially affect all three mechanisms of arrhythmias.

Automatic arrhythmias

Abnormal automaticity, whether atrial or ventricular, is generally seen in patients who are acutely ill and as a result have significant metabolic abnormalities. The metabolic abnormalities appear to change the characteristics of phase 4 of the cardiac action potential. The changes that most likely account for enhanced abnormal automaticity are an increased slope of phase 4 depolarization or a reduced maximum diastolic potential (i.e., reduced negativity in the transmembrane potential at the beginning of phase 4). Either type of change can cause the rapid, spontaneous generation of action potentials and thus precipitate inappropriate tachycardia (Figure 2.2).

An antiarrhythmic drug that might be effective against automatic tachyarrhythmias is likely to reduce one or both effects. Unfortunately, no drug has been shown to reliably improve abnormal automaticity in cardiac tissue. Therefore, the mainstay of therapy is to treat the underlying illness and reverse the metabolic abnormalities causing abnormal automaticity.

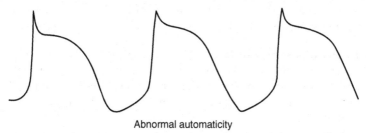

Abnormal automaticity

Figure 2.2 Abnormal automaticity causes rapid, spontaneous generation of action potentials and, thus, inappropriate tachycardia.

Triggered activity

Triggered arrhythmias, whether pause dependent (i.e., caused by early afterdepolarizations (EADs)) or catechol dependent (caused by delayed afterdepolarizations (DADs)), are related, as we have seen, to abnormal oscillations in the action potential. The precise mechanism of either type of afterdepolarization is only poorly understood, and no drug therapy is available that specifically eliminates the ionic fluxes responsible for EADs or DADs.

EADs are associated with prolongation of the action potential in susceptible individuals. A logical treatment, therefore, is to administer a drug that reduces the duration of the action potential. Although such antiarrhythmic drugs exist (Class IB drugs), their benefit in treating triggered arrhythmias caused by EADs has been spotty at best. Instead, as mentioned in Chapter 1, the best treatments devised for EAD-mediated tachyarrhythmias have endeavored to eliminate the offending agent and to increase the heart rate to remove the pauses necessary for the development of the arrhythmias. The major significance of antiarrhythmic drugs relative to EADs is that such drugs are a common *cause* of EADs.

Similarly, the best treatment devised for DADs does not address the specific ionic causes of DADs themselves. Treating the arrhythmias most often involves discontinuing digitalis and administering beta blockers.

Brugada syndrome
This syndrome is caused by abnormalities in the rapid sodium channel. Antiarrhythmic drugs that further block the sodium channel (Class I drugs) seem to potentiate the abnormalities associated with Brugada syndrome and should be avoided. Other drugs, including

beta blockers and amiodarone, have at best proven ineffective in treating this syndrome.

Reentrant arrhythmias

In contrast to the limited usefulness of antiarrhythmic drugs in treating automatic arrhythmias and channelopathies, these drugs, at least in theory, directly address the mechanism responsible for reentrant arrhythmias.

A functioning reentrant circuit requires a series of prerequisites—an anatomic or functional circuit must be present, one limb of the circuit must display slow conduction, and a second limb must display a prolonged refractory period (to produce unidirectional block). One can immediately grasp the potential benefit of a drug that, by changing the shape of the cardiac action potential, alters the conductivity and refractoriness of the tissues forming the reentrant circuit.

Figure 2.3 illustrates what might happen if a reentrant circuit were exposed to drugs. A drug that increases the duration of the cardiac action potential (thereby increasing refractory periods) further lengthens the already long refractory period of one pathway, and thus may convert unidirectional block to bidirectional block, which chemically amputates one of the pathways of the reentrant circuit. Alternatively, a drug that has the opposite effect on refractory periods—one that reduces the duration of the action potential and shortens refractory periods—may shorten the refractory period of one pathway so that the refractory periods of both pathways are relatively equal. Without a difference between the refractory periods of the two limbs of the circuit, reentry cannot be initiated.

The key point in understanding how drugs affect reentrant arrhythmias is that reentry requires a critical relationship between the refractory periods and the conduction velocities of the two limbs of the reentrant circuit. Because antiarrhythmic drugs can change these refractory periods and conduction velocities, the drugs can make reentrant arrhythmias less likely to occur.

Proarrhythmia

The manner in which antiarrhythmic drugs work against reentrant arrhythmias has an obvious negative implication. For example, if a patient with a previous myocardial infarction and asymptomatic, nonsustained ventricular tachycardia had an occult reentrant circuit whose electrophysiologic properties were not able to support a reentrant arrhythmia, such as the circuit shown in Figure 2.3b, the patient might be given a Class IIB drug (i.e., a drug that reduces the

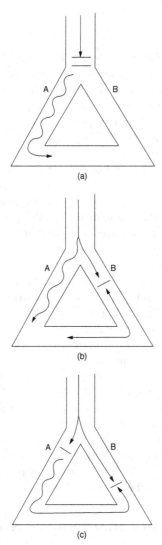

(a)

(b)

(c)

Figure 2.3 Effect of antiarrhythmic drugs on a reentrant circuit. (a) A prototypical reentrant circuit (see Figures 1.6 and 1.7). (b) Changes that might occur with the administration of a Class III drug such as sotalol that increases the duration of the cardiac action potential and thus increases refractory periods. With such a drug, the refractory period of pathway B may be sufficiently prolonged to prevent reentry from being initiated. (c) Changes that might occur with the administration of a drug such as lidocaine that shortens the duration of the action potential and of refractory periods. The refractory period of pathway B may be shortened to the extent that the refractory periods of pathways A and B become nearly equal. A premature impulse is likely to either conduct or block both pathways and thus prevent initiation of reentry.

action potential duration) to suppress the asymptomatic arrhythmia. Although it is possible that the drug will suppress the ambient ectopy, it is also possible that it might selectively reduce the refractory period of the pathway with the longer refractory period, thus giving this circuit the characteristics shown in Figure 2.3a. In other words, the drug might make a reentrant arrhythmia much more likely to occur.

Anytime an antiarrhythmic drug is given to a patient with a potential reentrant circuit, the drug may change the electrophysiologic characteristics of the circuit in such a way as to make a sustained arrhythmia either less likely or more likely to occur. Both outcomes are possible, and perhaps equally likely. Unfortunately, it is the very same mechanism that produces an antiarrhythmic effect that causes antiarrhythmic drugs to also produce a proarrhythmic effect. Proarrhythmia is therefore not a bizarre, inexplicable, idiosyncratic, or rare side effect of antiarrhythmic drugs. Proarrhythmia is an entirely predictable, inherent property of antiarrhythmic drugs. Since antiarrhythmia and proarrhythmia occur by the same mechanism, one cannot have one effect without the other.

Proarrhythmia is a fairly common occurrence, but it was only poorly recognized until the late 1980s. The failure to recognize that drug therapy may worsen arrhythmias often leads to inappropriate therapy (such as increasing or adding to the offending drug) and sometimes to death. Herein lies the problem in considering antiarrhythmic drugs to be "soothing balms."

Whether an antiarrhythmic drug will make an arrhythmia better or worse is usually difficult to predict before administering the drug. Therefore, proarrhythmia is a possibility for which one must be vigilant whenever these drugs are prescribed.

Classification of antiarrhythmic drugs

For any set of entities, a useful classification system is one that provides a relatively simple, logical framework that facilitates teaching and learning, aids in communication, allows practical generalizations, and offers insights into the essential nature of these entities. Two general classification schemes have been set forth for antiarrhythmic drugs—the Vaughan-Williams scheme, initially proposed in 1971, and the so-called Sicilian Gambit, proposed about 20 years later. Both systems are discussed briefly below. For the vast majority of clinicians, the older Vaughan-Williams system more nearly fulfills the essential purpose of a classification system.

Vaughan-Williams scheme

Until the late 1960s, so few antiarrhythmic drugs were available that no classification system was needed. When new drugs began to arrive with increasing frequency, however, several classification systems were proposed; the Vaughan-Williams scheme is the one proved to have the greatest practical value.

The Vaughan-Williams system (Table 2.1) is useful because it groups drugs according to their major mechanisms of action, that is, according to which channels they bind and block on the cardiac cell membrane. Thus, Class I drugs block the sodium channel (and thereby slow conduction velocity); Class II drugs block

Table 2.1 Vaughan-Williams classification system of antiarrhythmic drugs

---

Class I: Sodium-channel-blocking drugs
  Class IA: Moderately slow conduction and moderately prolong action potential
    duration
  Quinidine
  Procainamide
  Disopyramide
  Class IB: Minimally slow conduction and shorten action potential duration
  Lidocaine
  Mexiletine
  Tocainide
  Phenytoin
  Class IC: Markedly slow conduction and minimally prolong action potential
    duration
  Flecainide
  Encainide
  Propafenone
  Moricizine*
Class II: Beta-blocking drugs
Class III: Prolong action potential duration
  Amiodarone
  Sotalol
  Ibutilide
  Dofetilide
Class IV: Calcium-channel-blocking drugs

---

*Moricizine does not display the same affinity for the sodium channel as for other Class IC drugs, and some classify it as a IB drug. It is classified as a IC drug here to emphasize its proarrhythmic effects (which are only rarely seen with true Class IB drugs).

adrenergic receptors (and blunt the effect of sympathetic stimulation on cardiac electrophysiology); Class III drugs block potassium channels (and increase refractory periods); and Class IV drugs block calcium channels (and affect the areas of the heart that are depolarized primarily via calcium channels, i.e., the SA and AV nodes).

To take into account some of the obvious differences among the Class I drugs, the Vaughan-Williams system further subdivides these drugs into three subgroups: Class IA drugs—quinidine, procainamide, and disopyramide—slow conduction moderately (by slowing depolarization) and also moderately increase refractory periods (by increasing action potential duration); Class IB drugs—lidocaine, tocainide, mexiletine, and phenytoin—do not slow conduction and actually decrease the duration of the action potential; and Class IC drugs—flecainide, encainide, propafenone, and moricizine—produce a pronounced slowing of conduction velocity but very little prolongation of refractory periods.

By attempting to classify drugs according to their major membrane effects, the Vaughan-Williams scheme facilitates thinking about antiarrhythmic drugs in terms of their electrophysiologic properties. The prototypical electrophysiologic effects of the various classes of drugs are depicted in Figure 2.4.

Critics of this classification system point out that antiarrhythmic drugs often cause mixed effects on the cardiac cell and that antiarrhythmic drugs in the same Vaughan-Williams group can, clinically speaking, behave quite differently from one another. The most important confounding variable relates to how antiarrhythmic drugs affect sodium and potassium channels. In fact, the success of the Vaughan-Williams scheme hinges, to a large extent, on its ability to characterize the variable effects of Class I and Class III drugs on the sodium and potassium channels and, thus, on conduction velocities and refractory periods.

The binding characteristics of the sodium-blocking drugs, for instance, are complex. Although all Class I drugs bind to the sodium channel, they do not bind tonically (i.e., they do not "stick" to the channel). Instead, the drugs are constantly binding and unbinding from the sodium channel. Actual blockade of the sodium channel (and thus slowing of depolarization) occurs only if a drug is bound to the sodium channel at the time the channel first opens. However, many Class I drugs bind to the sodium channel only after it has already opened (i.e., when it is in the "activated" state). Thus, to

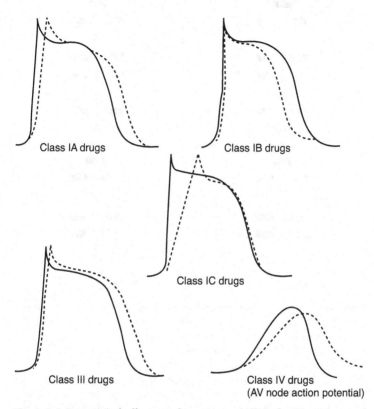

Class IA drugs

Class IB drugs

Class IC drugs

Class III drugs

Class IV drugs
(AV node action potential)

Figure 2.4 Prototypical effects on the action potential of various classes of antiarrhythmic drugs. The solid lines represent the baseline action potential; dotted lines represent the changes that result when various classes of antiarrhythmic drugs are given. The Purkinje fiber action potential is shown except in the case of Class IV drugs, for which the AV nodal action potential is depicted.

cause sodium-channel blockade, a Class I drug must first bind to an activated sodium channel and then stay bound to that channel until the channel reopens (at which time, block finally occurs). Therefore, the effect of a Class I drug on the sodium channel depends on its binding kinetics—the rate at which that drug binds to and unbinds from the sodium channel (or alternatively, its effect depends on how "sticky" the drug is once it binds to the channel; Figure 2.5). In the presence of "nonsticky" drugs that unbind rapidly (i.e., a drug with *rapid* binding kinetics), blockade of the sodium channel may be

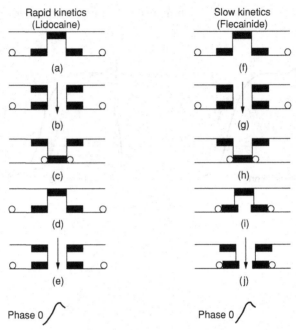

Figure 2.5 The effect of binding kinetics—the "stickiness" of a Class I drug—determines its effect on the sodium channel. As in Figure 2.1, the m and h gates are depicted; drugs are represented by open circles. Panels (a) through (e) illustrate the effect of lidocaine, a drug with rapid kinetics. (a) When lidocaine is first administered, it is not yet bound to the h gate. (b) The next time the cell is stimulated, the sodium channel functions normally. (c) However, once the h gate becomes activated, lidocaine binds to it. (Many Class I drugs bind only when the binding site is in the activated state, as the h gate is in this panel.) Because of the rapid unbinding of lidocaine, however, it quickly unbinds from the h gate. (d) Just before the next action potential is generated, lidocaine is no longer bound. (e) The next activation of the sodium channel therefore proceeds normally, and no slowing of conduction occurs. Panels (f) through (j) illustrate the effect of flecainide, a drug with slow kinetics. Panels (f) through (h) show reactions identical to those in panels (a) through (c). (f) When flecainide is first administered, it is not yet bound to the h gate. (g) The first activation of the sodium channel after flecainide is administered proceeds normally. (h) Flecainide, like lidocaine, first binds to the h gate as soon as that gate becomes activated. Unlike lidocaine, however, flecainide displays slow unbinding kinetics. (i) Just before the next action potential is generated, the drug is still attached to the h gate. (j) Thus, the h gate is partially closed when the sodium channel is next engaged, which leads to slow entry of sodium into the cell, a slow upstroke in the resultant action potential, and slowing of conduction velocity. At faster heart rates, drugs such as lidocaine have less time to unbind and can behave more like flecainide.

minimal. Drugs with rapid binding kinetics therefore produce relatively little reduction in conduction velocity. On the other hand, "sticky" drugs that unbind slowly (i.e., drugs that have *slow* binding kinetics) produce significant blockade of the sodium channels and thus substantially reduce conduction velocity. In general, the slower the binding kinetics of a sodium-blocking drug, the more effect the drug has on conduction velocity.

To further complicate the issue, the effect of Class I drugs on the sodium channel is partially situational. All Class I drugs, for instance, display *use dependence*: at faster heart rates, the sodium-channel block increases. Use dependence is simply a result of binding kinetics, which reflects that at faster heart rates, there is less time for the drug to unbind from the sodium channel before the next action potential begins; thus, at faster heart rates, the drugs have a more profound effect on conduction velocity than they have at slower heart rates. In addition, ischemia, hyperkalemia, and acidosis can slow the binding kinetics of Class I drugs and thus increase the effect of the drugs on the sodium channel. For instance, lidocaine, a Class IB drug with very rapid binding kinetics and thus little effect on conduction velocity in normal tissue, can have a profound effect on conduction velocity in ischemic tissue.

The Vaughan-Williams classification system accounts for the binding kinetics of the sodium-blocking drugs. Class IB drugs have very rapid sodium-channel-binding kinetics and, as noted, these drugs produce relatively little effect on conduction velocity. Class IC drugs have very slow binding kinetics and thus produce marked slowing of conduction velocity. The binding kinetics of Class IA drugs are intermediate, so these drugs have a moderate effect on conduction velocity. Although no classification system is likely to neatly characterize the nuances of sodium binding for every drug, the Vaughan-Williams system offers reasonably accurate generalizations about sodium-binding properties of antiarrhythmic drugs.

The Vaughan-Williams scheme is more challenged when one begins to consider the effect of antiarrhythmic drugs on the potassium channel. One of the basic premises of the Vaughan-Williams system is that Class I drugs bind the sodium channel and Class III drugs bind the potassium channel, but in fact many drugs have effects on both the sodium and potassium channels. As a result, application of the Vaughan-Williams system becomes very difficult in some cases. For instance, experts still disagree about whether moricizine rightly belongs to Class IB or Class IC. (The author holds with those who favor

Class IC, believing that the most remarkable clinical characteristic of moricizine is its robust Class-IC-like propensity to cause proarrhythmias.) Worse, amiodarone has properties from all four Vaughan-Williams classes. Ultimately, the classification of some drugs appears to be a matter of consensus rather than a matter of science.

Although the Vaughan-Williams scheme thus appears incapable of offering definitive classification for all possible mixtures of sodium- and potassium-channel blockade, it nonetheless suggests a framework for characterizing even difficult-to-classify drugs. The framework becomes apparent when one thinks of the general interplay of sodium-blocking and potassium-blocking properties as representing a continuum of possible effects instead of a categorical series of discrete effects (Figure 2.6). The advantage of thinking about drug effects along a continuum is that hard-to-classify drugs, such as moricizine and amiodarone, can be positioned at appropriate points along the continuum instead of being arbitrarily assigned to a specific class. In fact, the problem of classification is largely reduced to one of

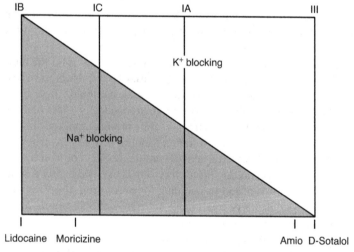

Figure 2.6 The sodium (Na^+)- and potassium (K^+)-blocking properties of antiarrhythmic drugs can be displayed as a continuum of effects. Class IB drugs can be viewed as having pure sodium-blocking effects and thus hold down the left side of the grid. Class III drugs can be viewed as having pure potassium-blocking effects and thus hold down the right side of the grid. The approximate positions of the Class IC and IA drugs are illustrated. Drugs that do not quite fit the classic Vaughan-Williams classification scheme (e.g., moricizine and amiodarone) can still be positioned appropriately along the grid.

Table 2.2 Clinical generalizations based on Vaughan-Williams class

Vaughan-Williams class	Location of activity	General level of efficacy	End-organ toxicity	Potential for proarrhythmia
Class IA	A, V	2+	3+	2+
Class IB	V	1+	1+	1+
Class IC	A, V	3+	1+	3+
Class II	AVN, V	1+	1+	0
Class III	A, V	2+ (amio 4+)	1+ (amio 4+)	2+ (amio 1+)
Class IV	AVN	1+	1+	0

A, atrium; amio, amiodarone; AVN, atrioventricular node; V, ventricle.

judging where on the continuum one class ends and the next begins (i.e., the problem becomes a matter of degree instead of a matter of kind). The Vaughan-Williams classification system, though admittedly imperfect, helps to locate drugs along the continuum, and therefore helps to elucidate the electrophysiologic properties even of drugs that are difficult to formally classify.

As it happens, the Vaughan-Williams scheme also allows one to make other clinically relevant generalizations about antiarrhythmic drugs. These generalizations, summarized in Table 2.2, relate to the types of arrhythmias that can be treated, the general level of efficacy and of therapy-limiting side effects, and the general risk of proarrhythmia associated with drugs within a class. (Class-specific features of antiarrhythmic drugs are discussed in Part 2 of this book.)

Sicilian Gambit scheme

In 1990, a group of eminent electrophysiologists retreated to Taormina, Sicily, to consider the issue of the classification of antiarrhythmic drugs because of the well-recognized limitations of the Vaughan-Williams scheme: the oversimplification of concepts about antiarrhythmic drugs, the common grouping of drugs with dissimilar actions, the inability to group certain drugs accurately, and the failure to take into account many actions of antiarrhythmic drugs that became recognized only long after the Vaughan-Williams system had been proposed. What emerged was a new approach to the classification of antiarrhythmic drugs; the inventors imaginatively named the approach the Sicilian Gambit.

The Vaughan-Williams scheme is based on whether drugs produce block in one or more of a few sites on the cell membrane, but the Sicilian Gambit takes into account a host of additional actions of antiarrhythmic drugs—the type and degree of blockade of channels, antagonistic and agonistic effects on receptors, effects on the sodium–potassium pump, the time constants of binding to cellular sites, effects on second messengers, and the affinity for binding on the basis of whether the cell is in an active or inactive state. The resultant schema is shown in Figure 2.7.

Drug	Channels					Receptors				Pumps	Clinical effects			Clinical effects	
	Na			Ca	k	α	β	M₂	A1	Na-k ATPase	Left ventricular function	Sinus Rate	Extra cardiac		
	Fast	Med	Slow												
Lidocaine	O										→	→	⊘		↓
Mexiletine	O										→	→	⊘		↓
Tocainide	O										→	→	●		↓
Moricizine	◑										↓	→	O	↑	
Procainamide		Ⓐ			⊘						↓	→	●	↑	↑ ↑
Disopyramide		Ⓐ			⊘			O			↓	→	⊘	↓↑	↑ ↑
Quinidine		Ⓐ			⊘	O		O			→	↓	⊘	↓↑	↑ ↑
Propafenone		Ⓐ					⊘				↓	↓	O	↑	↑
Flecainide			Ⓐ	O							↓	→	O	↑	↑ ↑
Encainide			Ⓐ								↓	→	O	↑	↑
Bepridil	O			●	⊘						?	↓	O		↑
Verapamil	O			●		⊘					↓	↓	O	↑	
Diltiazem				⊘							↓	↓	O	↑	
Bretylium					●	◪	◪				→	↓	O		↑
Sotalol					●		●				↓	↓	O	↑	↑
Amiodarone	O			O	●	⊘	⊘				→	↓	●	↑	↑
Alinidine				⊘	●						?	↓	●		
Nadolol							●				↓	↓	O	↑	
Propranolol	O						●				↓	↓	O	↑	
Atropine								●			→	↑	⊘	↓	
Adenosine									□		?	↓	O	↑	
Digoxin									□	●	↑	↓	●	↑	↓

Relative potency of block: O Low ⊘ Moderate ● High   A = Activated state blocker
□ = Agonist ◪ = Agonist/Antagonist   I = Inactivated state blocker

Figure 2.7 The Sicilian Gambit, a schema listing all major known properties of antiarrhythmic drugs. Effects of each drug on channels, receptors, and pumps are shown, as are some of the clinical effects. (Reproduced with permission from Members of the Sicilian Gambit. *Antiarrhythmic Therapy: A Pathophysiologic Approach.* Armonk, NY: Futura, 1994:94).

Two major differences exist between the Vaughan-Williams scheme and the Sicilian Gambit approach. First, the Sicilian Gambit is far more thorough than the Vaughan-Williams system in describing the precise actions of antiarrhythmic drugs. Second, inasmuch as each drug is essentially in its own class (since no two drugs are exactly alike in all the ways listed), the Sicilian Gambit is not a true classification system. Instead, it is a tabular list of virtually everything known about each drug.

This is not to say that the Sicilian Gambit is not useful. It is, in fact, useful to have a complete tabulation of all known effects of antiarrhythmic drugs. Such a table allows one to easily compare the recognized similarities and differences among drugs. Further, when the mechanisms of arrhythmias have become more precisely delineated, precise knowledge of individual drugs may help in formulating more accurate guesses as to effective pharmacologic therapy (which was a specific goal in devising the Sicilian Gambit), although it is likely to be always true that nearly identical patients with nearly identical arrhythmias often respond differently to the same drug. In addition, a tabulated system is certainly helpful to basic researchers.

However, because the Sicilian Gambit is not a true classification system, it does not offer much help to the average clinician in learning about or communicating about antiarrhythmic drugs. Nor does it aid in formulating practical generalizations about these drugs. Especially for the nonexpert, the Vaughan-Williams system, with all its limitations, remains the most useful means of categorizing antiarrhythmic drugs; it is the system that will be used throughout this book.

Part 2

Clinical features of
antiarrhythmic drugs

CHAPTER 3

Class I antiarrhythmic drugs

The feature that gains an antiarrhythmic drug admission into Class I is blockade of the rapid sodium channel. Yet, because of their varied effects on the sodium channel and the potassium channel, drugs assigned to Class I can behave very differently from one another. On the basis of their sodium and potassium effects, Class I drugs have been subclassified into groups IA, IB, and IC. The major clinical features, electrophysiologic properties, and adverse effects of Class I antiarrhythmic drugs are summarized in the accompanying tables.

Class IA

Class IA drugs can be thought of as all-purpose antiarrhythmic agents because they are moderately effective in treating most types of tachyarrhythmias. Unfortunately, they are also moderately effective in causing both major varieties of side effects—end-organ toxicity and proarrhythmias.

As shown in Figure 3.1, Class IA drugs block the rapid sodium channel (slowing the upstroke of the cardiac action potential and therefore slowing conduction velocity) and the potassium channel (prolonging the duration of the action potential and prolonging refractoriness). These electrophysiologic effects are manifested in both atrial and ventricular tissue, and therefore Class IA drugs have the potential of treating both atrial and ventricular tachyarrhythmias. The major clinical features of Class IA antiarrhythmic drugs are summarized in Table 3.1, and the major electrophysiologic features are summarized in Table 3.2.

Quinidine
Quinidine is the D-isomer of the antimalarial quinine, a drug that was noted to be effective in the treatment of palpitations as long

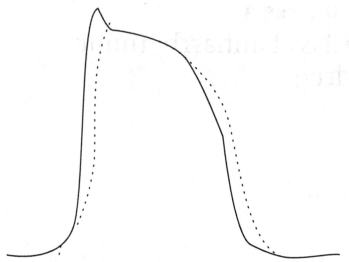

Figure 3.1 Effect of Class IA drugs on the cardiac action potential. Baseline action potential is displayed as a solid line; the dashed line indicates the effect of Class IA drugs.

ago as the eighteenth century. Quinidine itself was recognized as an effective antiarrhythmic agent in the early twentieth century.

Clinical pharmacology
Quinidine is administered orally as one of three salts (quinidine sulfate, quinidine gluconate, or quinidine polygalacturonate). All three forms of the drug have been made available because some patients tolerate one salt better than another. Approximately 80–90% of the sulfate preparation is absorbed after oral administration, and peak plasma concentrations are reached within 2 hours. The gluconate and polygalacturonate preparations are absorbed more slowly and less completely than the sulfate formulation. Quinidine is 80–90% protein bound in the circulation and has a large volume of distribution. The concentration of the drug is 4–10 times higher in the heart, liver, and kidneys than it is in the circulation. The drug is eliminated mainly through hepatic metabolism. Its elimination half-life is 5–8 hours but may be prolonged in patients with congestive heart failure or in the elderly.

Electrophysiologic effects
Quinidine blocks the sodium channel and slows the rate of depolarization of the action potential. Like all Class IA drugs, quinidine

Table 3.1 Clinical pharmacology of Class IA drugs

	Quinidine	Procainamide	Disopyramide
GI absorption	80–90%	70–90%	80–90%
Protein binding	80–90%	Weak	Variable (less binding at higher drug levels)
Elimination	Liver	Metabolized in liver to NAPA; PA and NAPA excreted by kidneys	60% kidneys 40% liver
Half-life	5–8 h	3–5 h	8–9 h
Therapeutic level	2–5 μg/mL	4–12 μg/mL (PA) 9–20 μg/mL (NAPA)	2–5 μg/mL
Dosage range	300–600 mg q6h (sulfate) 324–972 mg q6–8h (gluconate)	15 mg/kg IV, then 1–6 mg/min IV; or 500– 1250mg PO q6h	100–200 mg q6h

NAPA, *N*-acerylprocainamide; PA, procainamide.

binds and unbinds from the sodium channel more slowly than does lidocaine, but more rapidly than do Class IC agents. Thus, its effect on conduction velocity is midway between drugs in Class IB and IC. Its effects on the potassium channels result in prolongation of the action potential and, therefore, of the refractory period. These electrophysiologic effects are seen in both atrial and ventricular tissues. Quinidine can suppress automaticity in Purkinje fibers. Like all drugs that prolong refractoriness, quinidine can cause early afterdepolarizations (and thus torsades de pointes) in susceptible individuals.

Hemodynamic effects
Quinidine blocks the α-adrenergic receptors, which can lead to peripheral vasodilation and reflex sinus tachycardia. The effects tend to be minimal when the drug is given orally but can be profound with intravenous administration. Thus, the intravenous form of quinidine is used only rarely. Quinidine also has a vagolytic effect, which can manifest by improving conduction through the atrioventricular (AV)

Table 3.2 Electrophysiologic effects of Class IA drugs

	Quinidine	Procainamide	Disopyramide
Conduction velocity	Decrease ++	Decrease ++	Decrease ++
Refractory periods	Increase ++	Increase ++	Increase ++
Automaticity	Suppress +	Suppress +	Suppress +
Afterdepolarizations	May cause EADs	May cause EADs	May cause EADs
Efficacy			
Atrial fibrillation/atrial flutter	++	++	++
AVN reentry	+	+	+
Macroreentry	+	+	+
PVCs	++	++	++
VT/VF	++	++	++

AVN, AV node; EADs, early afterdepolarizations; PVCs, premature ventricular complexes; VT/VF, ventricular tachycardia and ventricular fibrillation.

node. The vagolytic effect is important clinically when treating atrial fibrillation or atrial flutter; enhanced AV nodal conduction caused by quinidine can lead to a more rapid ventricular response, unless AV nodal blocking agents are also given. No significant myocardial depression occurs with quinidine.

Therapeutic uses
Quinidine is moderately effective in treating both atrial and ventricular tachyarrhythmias. Approximately 50% of patients treated with quinidine for atrial fibrillation remain in sinus rhythm after 1 year. Quinidine acts on the accessory pathway in patients with bypass-tract-mediated tachycardias and on the fast pathway in patients with AV nodal reentrant tachycardia. Thus, quinidine has

been used to treat virtually all varieties of reentrant supraventricular tachyarrhythmias.

Quinidine is effective in suppressing premature ventricular complexes and nonsustained ventricular tachycardias, but because of the proarrhythmic potential of quinidine (and most other antiarrhythmic agents), these arrhythmias should not be treated except to suppress significant symptoms. For the same reason, quinidine should not be used to treat sustained ventricular tachycardia without the protection of an implantable defibrillator.

Adverse effects and interactions

Symptomatic side effects occur in 30–50% of patients taking quinidine, and the drug must be discontinued in 20–30% of patients because of toxicity. The most common side effects are gastrointestinal, mainly diarrhea. In general, if diarrhea occurs, the drug should be discontinued, because the diarrhea is usually not adequately controlled with medication and the resultant electrolyte imbalances may exacerbate the very arrhythmias that are being treated. Quinidine can also cause dizziness, headache, or cinchonism (tinnitus, visual blurring, and hearing disturbances). Rashes are fairly common, and significant hypersensitivity reactions such as hemolytic anemia and thrombocytopenia can also occur. Lupus and hepatitis have also been reported with the drug.

As is the case with all Class IA drugs, proarrhythmia is a major consideration any time quinidine is used. Any drug that prolongs the duration of the action potential can produce torsades de pointes in susceptible individuals, and any drug that alters conduction velocity or refractoriness can exacerbate reentrant arrhythmias. Quinidine thus can (and does) cause ventricular arrhythmias by either of these mechanisms. Quinidine-induced syncope was recognized decades ago, but it was only relatively recently that this clinical syndrome was shown to be caused by ventricular tachyarrhythmias. Quinidine-induced ventricular arrhythmias often occur early, usually within 3–5 days after the drug is begun, but can be seen at any time. Although the incidence of quinidine-induced proarrhythmia is difficult to quantify, a meta-analysis of randomized trials using quinidine to treat atrial fibrillation indicated a total mortality of 2.9% in patients receiving quinidine, compared with a mortality of 0.8% in patients receiving placebo. This excess mortality is likely due to proarrhythmia. Because of the risk of proarrhythmia, doctors should strongly consider placing patients on a cardiac monitor for several days when treatment with quinidine is elected.

Several relevant drug interactions have been reported with quinidine. Quinidine potentiates the effect of anticholinergics, warfarin, and phenothiazines. Increased digoxin levels routinely occur when quinidine is given to patients taking digoxin. Quinidine levels are decreased by phenobarbital, rifampin, and phenytoin; they are increased by amiodarone.

Procainamide

Procainamide came into clinical use in 1951. Its availability in both oral and intravenous forms made it an attractive drug for many years in the treatment of both acute and chronic tachyarrhythmias.

Clinical pharmacology

When given intravenously, procainamide's onset of action is almost immediate; after oral intake, the onset of action is approximately 1 hour. Absorption after oral intake is 70–90%, and the drug is only weakly protein bound. Fifty percent of the drug is excreted in the urine, and variable amounts of procainamide are metabolized by the liver, by the process of acetylation, to N-acetylprocainamide (NAPA), an active metabolite with Class III antiarrhythmic properties. The amount of NAPA in the plasma depends on hepatic function and the acetylator phenotype. (Approximately 50% of the population is "slow acetylator," and these individuals may be more susceptible to procainamide-induced lupus.) Both the parent compound and NAPA are excreted by the kidneys. The elimination half-life is 3–5 hours in normal individuals. Assays for measuring plasma levels of both procainamide and NAPA are readily available.

Dosage

Intravenous loading of procainamide should be given no more rapidly than 50 mg/min to minimize hemodynamic side effects, to a total dose of 15 mg/kg. Administration should be slowed if hypotension occurs and should be stopped if the QRS interval increases by more than 50% or if heart block occurs. A maintenance infusion of 1–6 mg/min can be used to maintain therapeutic levels. By oral administration, 3–6 g/day are usually given in divided doses. With currently available long-acting preparations, procainamide can be given every 6–12 hours. Because of its short half-life, administration every 3–4 hours is required with short-acting preparations.

Electrophysiologic effects
The electrophysiologic effects of procainamide are similar to those of quinidine.

Hemodynamic effects
Like quinidine, procainamide causes arteriolar vasodilation, an effect that is seen almost exclusively when the drug is given intravenously. This side effect is easier to control with procainamide than with quinidine by titrating the infusion rate. Procainamide has an anticholinergic effect but it is of less magnitude than that of quinidine. Negative inotropic effects are negligible unless toxic levels of the drug are reached, especially when NAPA levels exceed 30 μg/mL.

Therapeutic uses
The therapeutic uses of procainamide are similar to those of quinidine. The drug can be used for all varieties of reentrant atrial and ventricular arrhythmias, and its overall efficacy for both atrial and ventricular tachyarrhythmias is similar to that of quinidine. Because procainamide is available for relatively rapid intravenous loading, it has often been used to treat atrial fibrillation with rapid conduction down a bypass tract. Procainamide is also used for the acute conversion of atrial fibrillation and atrial flutter and to terminate or slow incessant ventricular tachycardias.

Adverse effects and interactions
Side effects that occur soon after beginning therapy with procainamide include hypotension (when the drug is administered intravenously) and gastrointestinal problems (especially nausea, vomiting, and diarrhea) in up to 25% of patients treated. With chronic administration of procainamide, agranulocytosis is the most serious problem. The problem is rare but carries a mortality as high as 25%. Agranulocytosis is usually seen within the first 3 months of therapy. Procainamide-induced lupus occurs in 20% of patients who take the drug chronically, and may be manifested by fever, rash, arthritis, pleuritis, or pericarditis. Symptoms usually (but not always) resolve within a few weeks of discontinuing the drug. Persistent fever due to procainamide, without any other manifestations of lupus, can also be seen. Procainamide-induced psychosis has also been reported.

Procainamide levels may be increased when the drug is given with amiodarone, trimethoprim, and especially cimetidine (but not ranitidine). Alcohol can decrease procainamide levels by increasing hepatic metabolism.

The cautions relative to proarrhythmia are the same for procainamide as those for quinidine.

Disopyramide
Disopyramide is chemically dissimilar to quinidine and procainamide but has virtually the same electrophysiologic effects. Disopyramide was approved for clinical use by the United States Food and Drug Administration (FDA) in 1977.

Clinical pharmacology
Disopyramide is an oral agent. Absorption is high (80–90%), and peak blood levels occur 2–3 hours after administration. Protein binding of the drug depends on its plasma concentration—at higher blood levels, less of the drug is bound; thus, toxicity is especially significant at these higher drug levels. Approximately 60% of the drug is excreted by the kidneys, and 40% is metabolized in the liver. Its major metabolite (an alkylated compound) has significant anticholinergic properties. The elimination half-life is 8–9 hours in normal individuals.

Dosage
The usual dosage of disopyramide is 100–200 mg every 6 hours. A longer-acting form given 200–300 mg every 12 hours is also available. The dosage should be adjusted downward in the presence of either hepatic or renal insufficiency.

Electrophysiologic effects
The electrophysiologic effects of disopyramide are similar to those of quinidine. In addition, disopyramide has significant anticholinergic effects, which can increase the sinus rate and enhance AV nodal conduction.

Hemodynamic effects
Disopyramide has a strong negative inotropic effect and should not be used in patients with depressed myocardial function, especially in patients with a history of congestive heart failure (more than 50% of whom have acute hemodynamic decompensation after administration of disopyramide).

Therapeutic uses

The therapeutic profile of disopyramide is very similar to that of quinidine. Its clinical usefulness, however, has been limited by its negative inotropic potential and its relatively strong anticholinergic properties. Aside from treating arrhythmias, disopyramide has also been reported to be effective in some patients with cardioneurogenic (vasovagal) syncope, presumably because its negative inotropic effects can delay the recruitment of cardiac C fibers (one of the afferent pathways that can stimulate the vasodepressor region of the medulla).

Adverse effects and interactions

The major adverse effects of disopyramide are related to myocardial depression and anticholinergic side effects. Disopyramide should not be used in patients with any degree of ventricular dysfunction, especially if they have a history of congestive heart failure. Symptoms of dry mouth, eyes, nose, and throat occur in as much as 40% of patients taking disopyramide. Urinary difficulty or urinary retention are significant problems with disopyramide in men older than 50 years but can also be seen in women. The drug can precipitate closed-angle glaucoma and should not be used in patients with a family history of glaucoma. Disopyramide can also produce hypoglycemia in occasional patients, apparently by increasing insulin levels.

Proarrhythmic effects of disopyramide are similar to those of quinidine.

Drug interactions include the decreasing of plasma disopyramide levels by phenobarbital, phenytoin, and rifampin. Other drugs with negative inotropic effects can exacerbate the myocardial depression seen with disopyramide.

Class IB

Class IB drugs are moderately useful in treating ventricular arrhythmias. Their major advantage is that, in marked contrast to the other Class I drugs, they have a low potential for causing proarrhythmia.

As shown in Figure 3.2, Class IB drugs have relatively little effect on the rapid sodium channel at normal heart rates and at therapeutic serum concentrations, so they have little effect on conduction velocity. Their major electrophysiologic effect is to decrease the duration

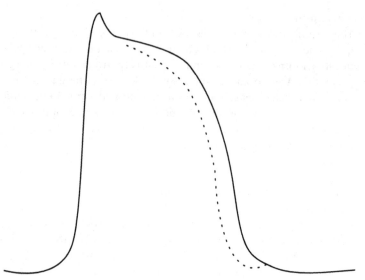

Figure 3.2 Effect of Class IB drugs on the cardiac action potential. Baseline action potential is displayed as a solid line; the dashed line indicates the effect of Class IB drugs.

of the action potential and, therefore, to decrease refractory periods. Probably because the duration of the action potential in atrial tissue is already shorter than that of ventricular tissue, Class IB drugs have little effect on atrial tissue and thus are useful only in the treatment of ventricular arrhythmias. Tables 3.3 and 3.4 summarize the major clinical features and electrophysiologic properties of Class IB antiarrhythmic drugs.

Lidocaine
Lidocaine has been used clinically since 1943 when it was introduced as a local anesthetic agent. In the 1950s, it gradually came into use for the acute treatment of ventricular arrhythmias, and it remains the drug of first choice for ventricular arrhythmias in many acute situations.

Clinical pharmacology
Although lidocaine is well absorbed in the gut, it is subject to extensive first-pass metabolism in the liver, so it is normally administered

Table 3.3 Clinical pharmacology of Class IB drugs

	Lidocaine	Mexiletine	Phenytoin
GI absorption	—	>90%	Variable
Protein binding	70%	70%	90%
Elimination	Liver	Liver	Liver
Half-life	1–4 h	8–16 h	24 h
Therapeutic level	1.5–5 μg/mL	0.75–2 μg/mL	10–20 μg/mL
Dosage range	1.5 mg/kg IV, then 1– 4 mg/min; repeat $^1/_2$ initial dose after 10 min	150–200 mg q8h	Oral: 300–500 mg/day in divided doses; IV loading: 7.5–10 mg at rate of 50 mg every 2 min

intravenously. Very little of the drug is excreted by the kidneys even after intravenous administration. Lidocaine is 70% bound to protein in plasma. Further, the proteins that bind lidocaine are acute-phase reactants; that is, during periods of stress, such as acute myocardial infarction, the proteins that bind lidocaine increase in plasma. Increased plasma binding during stress can prolong the elimination half-life from 1 or 2 hours to as long as 4 hours, and thus can cause lidocaine levels to increase even during a constant infusion.

Dosage

Lidocaine is generally loaded acutely by giving 1.5 mg/kg intravenously and initiating a constant infusion of 1–4 mg/min. When lidocaine is given acutely, it is rapidly distributed to the target organs (phase 1 distribution), but within 20 minutes, it is distributed throughout the rest of the body (phase 2 distribution); the initial immediate efficacy of the drug falls off during phase 2. Thus, two or three additional boluses are usually given at 10-minute intervals after the original bolus; the dosage of the additional boluses is usually half that of the initial bolus.

Table 3.4 Electrophysiologic effects of Class IB drugs

	Lidocaine	Mexiletine	Phenytoin
Conduction velocity	–	–	–
Refractory periods	Decrease +	Decrease +	Decrease +
Automaticity	Suppress ++	Suppress ++	Suppress ++
Afterdepolarizations	Suppresses EADs and DADs +	Suppresses DADs +	Suppresses DADs +
Efficacy			
Atrial fibrillation/atrial flutter	–	–	–
AVN reentry	–	–	–
Macroreentry	+/–	–	–
PVCs	++	++	+
VT/VF	+	+	+

AVN, AV node; EADs, early afterdepolarizations; DADs, delayed afterdepolarizations; PVCs, premature ventricular complexes; VT/VF, ventricular tachycardia and ventricular fibrillation.

Electrophysiologic effects

Typical of Class IB drugs, lidocaine (mainly because of its rapid binding kinetics) causes no slowing of the depolarization phase of the action potential and no slowing in conduction velocity in normal tissue. However, at fast heart rates or during ischemia, hypokalemia, or acidosis, lidocaine can substantially slow depolarization and conduction velocity. The duration of the action potential and the refractory period are shortened by lidocaine in ventricular tissue but not in atrial tissue. Lidocaine can suppress both normal and abnormal automaticity, which can lead to asystole when lidocaine is given in the setting of a ventricular escape rhythm. Lidocaine can also suppress early and late afterdepolarizations.

Hemodynamic effects
Lidocaine has little or no hemodynamic effect.

Therapeutic uses
Lidocaine is effective for ventricular tachyarrhythmias and is often the drug of choice for the emergent therapy of these arrhythmias because therapeutic plasma levels can be obtained rapidly. The drug has been shown to decrease the incidence of ventricular fibrillation in the setting of acute myocardial infarction but does not improve mortality.

Adverse effects and interactions
The predominant side effects relate to the central nervous system. Slurred speech, dizziness, perioral numbness and paresthesias, seizures, and respiratory arrest can all occur and are generally associated with toxic plasma levels.

Other drugs may affect plasma levels of lidocaine. Propranolol, metoprolol, and cimetidine (but not ranitidine) decrease hepatic blood flow and result in increased levels of lidocaine. Phenobarbital decreases plasma concentrations of lidocaine.

Lidocaine causes proarrhythmia only rarely.

Mexiletine
Mexiletine is an orally administered congener of lidocaine and was approved by the FDA in 1986.

Clinical pharmacology
Mexiletine is nearly completely absorbed from the gut and displays minimal first-pass hepatic clearance. Peak plasma levels occur in 4–6 hours, and the drug is approximately 70% protein bound. The drug is mainly metabolized by the liver, and the elimination half-life is from 8 to 16 hours.

Dosage
Because of the variable metabolism and because therapeutic and toxic doses of mexiletine tend to overlap, dosage must be individualized. Generally, unless hepatic disease is present, 150 mg is given every 8 hours. If there is no response after several days (at least 3 days) and if toxicity is not present, dosage can be increased to 200 mg every 8 hours. Dosage can be further increased after several

more days unless toxicity is present, but rarely can more than 750 mg/day be administered without significant side effects.

Electrophysiologic effects
The electrophysiologic effects of mexiletine are virtually identical to those of lidocaine.

Hemodynamic effects
Mexiletine has little or no effect on blood pressure or cardiac function.

Therapeutic uses
The therapeutic profile of mexiletine is similar to that of lidocaine; that is, it effectively suppresses ventricular arrhythmias. Unlike lidocaine, however, mexiletine is not particularly suitable for the treatment of emergent or acute arrhythmias because titrating the drug to an effective dose may take many days. Its use has, thus, been limited to treating chronic ventricular arrhythmias. Although mexiletine is effective in suppressing premature ventricular complexes and nonsustained ventricular tachycardia, these arrhythmias should generally not be treated unless they are producing significant symptoms. On the basis of serial drug testing in the electrophysiology laboratory, mexiletine rarely suppresses inducible sustained ventricular tachycardia; the drug is estimated to be effective for such suppression in only 5–10% of patients tested.

Adverse effects and interactions
As with lidocaine, central nervous system side effects predominate; tremor, blurred vision, and ataxia are the most common effects. Gastrointestinal symptoms are also common. While the drug generally has no hemodynamic effects, it has been reported to worsen heart failure in patients with severe cardiomyopathy. The drug has also been reported to cause thrombocytopenia.

Mexiletine levels can be reduced by phenytoin, phenobarbitol, and rifampin. Mexiletine levels can be increased by cimetidine, chloramphenicol, and isoniazid. Theophylline levels can be increased substantially when the drug is given with mexiletine. The side effects of mexiletine and lidocaine can be additive.

Typical of Class IB antiarrhythmic drugs, mexiletine displays only rare proarrhythmic effects.

Tocainide

Tocainide is another oral analog of lidocaine. Its properties are very similar to mexiletine, except that it is eliminated from the system by both the liver and the kidneys. Because tocainide was found to cause agranulocytosis in a small but substantial subset of patients exposed to the drug, it is essentially no longer used clinically except for the extraordinarily rare patient who needs a Class IB drug chronically but who cannot tolerate other drugs in this class.

Phenytoin

Phenytoin came into clinical use as an anticonvulsant in 1938. By the early 1950s, the drug was recognized to have antiarrhythmic properties. The drug enjoyed brief popularity as an antiarrhythmic agent in the early 1960s but was almost entirely supplanted when lidocaine and procainamide came into widespread use. Phenytoin has never been approved by the FDA for treating cardiac arrhythmias, and while in general phenytoin is not widely thought of as an antiarrhythmic agent, it can occasionally be quite useful for this purpose.

Clinical pharmacology

Phenytoin's oral absorption is relatively slow and highly variable. Peak serum levels can occur from 3 to 12 hours after an oral dose. The drug is 90% protein bound and is metabolized by the liver to inactive compounds. At lower plasma levels (<10 $\mu g/mL$), elimination is exponential. At higher plasma levels, elimination is dose dependent, and plasma levels increase disproportionately as dosage is increased. The average elimination half-life is 24 hours, but this value is highly variable.

Dosage

A drug-loading regimen is usually recommended with oral administration of phenytoin, especially if therapeutic levels are desired within 24 hours. Generally, 15 mg/kg is given orally in divided doses on day 1, followed by 7.5 mg/kg on day 2, followed by a maintenance dosage of 5 mg/kg on subsequent days (usually 300–500 mg/day in two or three divided doses). Chronic dosage should not be changed more often than at 10- to 14-day intervals because of the dose-dependent elimination of the drug.

Phenytoin can also be administered intravenously, preferably through a central intravenous line because of the tendency to produce phlebitis. As much as 50 mg/min can be given intravenously to a total dose of 7.5–10 mg/kg. Monitoring for the appearance of lateral gaze nystagmus during administration of the drug can be a useful indicator of therapeutic serum levels (10–20 μg/mL).

Electrophysiologic effects
The electrophysiologic profile of phenytoin is similar to that of lidocaine; it displays a rate-dependent effect on the sodium channel with rapid binding-unbinding characteristics. Thus, conduction velocity is minimally affected in normal tissue and at normal heart rates. Unlike other Class IB drugs, phenytoin also displays a centrally mediated antiadrenergic effect. Delayed afterdepolarizations of the type seen with digitalis toxicity are suppressed by phenytoin.

Hemodynamic effects
With rapid intravenous loading, hypotension can occur but can be controlled by titrating the rate of drug administration. Hypotension does not occur with oral administration. Phenytoin has no negative inotropic effects.

Therapeutic uses
Phenytoin is effective for ventricular tachyarrhythmias caused by digitalis toxicity, most likely because it suppresses delayed afterdepolarizations. In addition, because of its Class IB effects, phenytoin is occasionally effective in suppressing inducible sustained ventricular tachycardias in the electrophysiology laboratory (10–12% of the time). Phenytoin has also been moderately effective in suppressing ventricular arrhythmias in intensive care unit (ICU) settings in which enhanced automaticity is often invoked as an arrhythmic mechanism (ICU arrhythmias).

Adverse effects and interactions
The most common side effects involve the gastrointestinal and central nervous systems. Central nervous system symptoms (mainly ataxia and nystagmus) are related to plasma levels. Other less common side effects include osteomalacia (from interference with vitamin D metabolism), megaloblastic anemia (from interference with folate metabolism), and hypersensitivity reactions such as lupus, hepatic necrosis, hematologic disorders, and pseudolymphoma. Gingival hyperplasia, said to occur in up to 20% of children taking phenytoin, appears to be relatively rare in adults.

Several drug interactions have been seen with phenytoin. Phenytoin increases plasma levels of theophylline, quinidine, disopyramide, lidocaine, and mexiletine. Phenytoin levels are increased by cimetidine, isoniazid, sulfonamides, and amiodarone. Plasma levels of phenytoin can be reduced by theophylline. Like other Class IB drugs, phenytoin rarely causes proarrhythmia.

Class IC

Class IC drugs generated much excitement in the early to late 1980s because they are very effective in suppressing both atrial and ventricular tachyarrhythmias and generally cause only mild end-organ toxicity. When the proarrhythmic potential of Class IC drugs was more fully appreciated, however, the drugs quickly fell out of favor and one (encainide) was taken off the market entirely.

As shown in Figure 3.3, Class IC drugs have a relatively pronounced effect on the rapid sodium channel because of their slow sodium-channel-binding kinetics. Thus, they significantly slow conduction velocity even at normal heart rates. They have only a modest effect on repolarization. Class IC drugs have similar effects on

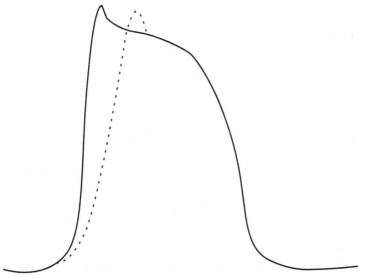

Figure 3.3 Effect of Class IC drugs on the cardiac action potential. Baseline action potential is displayed as a solid line; the dashed line indicates the effect of Class IC drugs.

Table 3.5 Clinical pharmacology of Class IC drugs

	Flecainide	Propafenone	Moricizine
GI absorption	>90%	>90%	>90%
Protein binding	40%	90%	>90%
Elimination	70% liver 30% kidneys	Liver	Liver (metabolized to >2 dozen compounds)
Half-life	12–24 h	6–7 h	Variable; usually 3–12 h
Therapeutic level	0.2–1.0 μg/mL	0.2–1.0 μg/mL	—
Dosage range	100–200 mg q12h	150–300 mg q8h	200–300 mg q8h

both atrial and ventricular tissue and are useful for both atrial and ventricular tachyarrhythmias. The major clinical features of Class IC antiarrhythmic drugs are summarized in Table 3.5, and the major electrophysiologic properties are shown in Table 3.6.

Flecainide
Flecainide was synthesized in 1972 and approved by the FDA in 1984.

Clinical pharmacology
Flecainide is well absorbed from the gastrointestinal tract, and peak plasma levels are reached 2–4 hours after an oral dose. Forty percent of the drug is protein bound. The drug is mainly metabolized by the liver (70%), but 30% is excreted unchanged by the kidneys. Flecainide has a long elimination half-life (12–24 h), so a steady state is not reached for 3–5 days after a change in oral dosage.

Dosage
The usual dosage is 100–400 mg/day orally, in divided doses. Generally, the beginning dosage is 100 mg every 12 hours. Dosage can be increased by 50 mg/dose (at 3- to 5-day intervals) to a maximal dosage of 200 mg every 12 hours.

Table 3.6 Electrophysiologic effects of Class IC drugs

	Flecainide	Propafenone	Moricizine
Conduction velocity	Decrease $+++$	Decrease $+++$	Decrease $++$
Refractory periods	No change (may lengthen RP in atrium)	No change	Decrease $+$
Automaticity	–	Suppresses	Suppresses
Afterdepolarizations	–	–	Suppresses EADs and DADs
Efficacy			
Atrial fibrillation/atrial flutter	$++$	$++$	$+$
AVN reentry	$++$	$++$	$+$
Macroreentry	$++$	$++$	$+$
PVCs	$+++$	$+++$	$++$
VT/VF	$++$	$++$	$++$

AVN, AV node; EADs, early afterdepolarizations; DADs, delayed afterdepolarizations; RP, refractory periods; PVCs, premature ventricular complexes; VT/VF, ventricular tachycardia and ventricular fibrillation.

Electrophysiologic effects

The major electrophysiologic feature of flecainide is a substantial slowing in conduction velocity. The prolonged slowing is directly related to the prolonged binding-unbinding time (i.e., the slow binding kinetics) of the drug. Although most Class IA agents have binding times in the range of 5 seconds, and Class IB drugs have binding times of approximately 0.3 seconds, flecainide has a binding time of 30 seconds. Thus, flecainide is virtually continuously bound to the sodium channel, and therefore produces slow conduction even at low heart rates (i.e., at rest). Flecainide subsequently has a dose-dependent effect on the electrocardiogram, manifested by a progressive prolongation of the PR and QRS intervals (reflecting its slowing of conduction velocity), with only a minor effect on the QT interval (reflecting its minimal effect on refractory periods). The drug depresses conduction in all areas of the heart.

Hemodynamic effects

Flecainide has a pronounced negative inotropic effect similar to that of disopyramide. The drug should not be given to patients with a history of congestive heart failure or with significantly depressed left ventricular ejection fraction.

Therapeutic uses

As one might predict from the universal nature of the drug's electrophysiologic properties, flecainide has an effect on both atrial and ventricular tachyarrhythmias. It has been shown to be effective for terminating and preventing atrial fibrillation and atrial flutter; if the arrhythmias recur, flecainide can slow the ventricular response. Because it affects accessory pathway function, flecainide is useful in the treatment of bypass-tract-mediated tachyarrhythmias. The drug has a profound suppressive effect on premature ventricular complexes and nonsustained ventricular tachycardia. It has been reported to suppress approximately 20–25% of inducible sustained ventricular tachycardias in the electrophysiology laboratory.

Flecainide is unsurpassed in suppressing premature ventricular complexes and nonsustained ventricular tachycardias, but it should not be used for this indication in patients who have underlying heart disease. This finding was made apparent by results of the Cardiac Arrhythmia Suppression Trial (CAST [1]), which tested the proposition that suppression of ventricular ectopy after myocardial infarction would reduce mortality. Patients receiving flecainide or encainide in this trial had significantly higher mortality rates than did patients receiving placebo. The significant difference in mortality has been attributed to the proarrhythmic properties of the Class IC drugs.

Adverse effects and interactions

Flecainide is generally better tolerated than most antiarrhythmic agents. Mild-to-moderate visual disturbances are the most common side effect, usually manifesting as blurred vision. Occasionally, gastrointestinal symptoms occur. However, no significant organ toxicity has been reported.

By far the most serious adverse effect of flecainide (and of all Class IC drugs) is its significant proarrhythmic potential (see the comparison to other Class I drugs in Table 3.7). Proarrhythmia with IC agents takes the form of exacerbation of reentrant ventricular tachycardia; torsades de pointes is not seen. Thus, the risk of proarrhythmia with flecainide is mainly limited to patients who have the potential for developing reentrant ventricular arrhythmias, that is, patients with underlying cardiac disease. CAST revealed that proarrhythmia with Class IC drugs is especially likely during times of acute myocardial ischemia. It is likely that ischemia potentiates the effect of these drugs just as it does with both Class IA and IB drugs. In any case, flecainide and other Class IC drugs appear to have a tendency to convert an episode of angina to an episode of sudden death. Class IC drugs should be avoided in patients with known or suspected coronary artery disease.

Flecainide levels may be increased by amiodarone, cimetidine, propranolol, and quinidine. Flecainide may modestly increase digoxin levels.

Encainide
Encainide is a Class IC drug whose electrophysiologic and clinical properties are very similar to those of flecainide. Encainide was removed from the market after CAST and is no longer available.

Propafenone
Propafenone was developed in the late 1960s and released for use in the United States in 1989.

Clinical pharmacology
Propafenone is well absorbed from the gastrointestinal tract and achieves peak blood levels 2–3 hours after an oral dose. It is subject to extensive first-pass hepatic metabolism that results in nonlinear kinetics—as the dosage of the drug is increased, hepatic metabolism becomes saturated; thus, a relatively small increase in dosage can produce a relatively large increase in drug levels. The drug is 90% protein bound and is metabolized by the liver. The elimination half-life is 6 or 7 hours after a steady state is reached. Generally, 3 days at a stable drug dosage achieves steady-state blood levels.

Table 3.7 Common adverse effects of Class I drugs

		Proarrhythmia	
	General toxicity	Reentrant VT	Torsades de pointes
Quinidine	GI (diarrhea), cinchonism, rashes, hemolytic anemia, and thrombocytopenia	++	++
Procainamide	Hypotension (IV), lupus, GI (nausea), and agranulocytosis	++	++
Disopyramide	Cardiac decompensation, urinary retention, and dry mouth and eyes	++	++
Lidocaine	CNS (slurred speech, paresthesias, and seizures)	+	−
Mexiletine	GI (nausea) and CNS (tremor and ataxia)	+	−
Phenytoin	GI (nausea), CNS (ataxia and nystagmus), hypersensitivity reactions (rashes and hematologic), osteomalacia, and megaloblastic anemia	+	−
Flecainide	Visual disturbances, GI (nausea), and cardiac decompensation	+++	−
Propafenone	GI (nausea), CNS (dizziness and ataxia), and cardiac decompensation (uncommon)	+++	−
Moricizine	Dizziness, headache, and nausea	++	−

Dosage

The usual dosage of propafenone is 150–300 mg every 8 hours. Generally, the beginning dosage is 150 mg or 225 mg every 8 hours. Dosage may be increased, but not more often than every third day.

Electrophysiologic effects

Propafenone produces potent blockade of the sodium channel, similar to other Class IC drugs. Unlike other Class IC agents, however, propafenone also causes a slight increase in the refractory periods of all cardiac tissue. In addition, propafenone has mild beta-blocking and calcium-blocking properties.

Hemodynamic effects

Propafenone has a negative inotropic effect that is relatively mild, substantially less than that seen with disopyramide or flecainide. The drug also blunts the heart rate during exercise. Both effects may be a result of its beta-blocking (and perhaps its calcium-blocking) properties.

Therapeutic uses

Like all Class IC agents, propafenone is effective in treating a wide variety of atrial and ventricular arrhythmias. Its therapeutic profile is similar to that of flecainide.

Adverse effects and interactions

The most common side effects of propafenone are dizziness, light-headedness, ataxia, nausea, and a metallic aftertaste. Exacerbation of congestive heart failure can be seen, especially in patients with histories of heart failure. Propafenone can cause a lupuslike facial rash, and also a condition called exanthematous pustulosis, which is a nasty rash accompanied by fever and a high white-blood-cell count. Generally, propafenone tends to cause more side effects than other Class IC antiarrhythmic drugs.

As is the case with all Class IC drugs, proarrhythmia is a significant problem with propafenone, but the problem is limited to patients with underlying heart disease. Most clinicians believe, and some clinical trials appear to show, that proarrhythmia with propafenone is somewhat less frequent than it is with flecainide.

Numerous drug interactions have been reported with propafenone. Phenobarbital, phenytoin, and rifampin decrease levels of propafenone. Quinidine and cimetidine increase levels of propafenone. Propafenone increases levels of digoxin, propranolol, metoprolol, theophylline, cyclosporine, and desipramine. It increases the effect of warfarin.

Moricizine

Moricizine, a phenothiazine derivative, has been in use in Russia since the 1970s. It was approved by the FDA in 1990.

Clinical pharmacology

Moricizine is absorbed almost completely when administered orally, and peak plasma levels occur within 1–2 hours. Moricizine is extensively metabolized in the liver to a multitude of compounds, some of which may have electrophysiologic effects. The elimination half-life of the parent compound is variable (generally, 3–12 h), but the half-life of some of its metabolites is substantially longer. Plasma levels of moricizine have not reflected the efficacy of the drug.

Dosage

Moricizine is usually initiated in dosages of 200 mg orally every 8 hours and may be increased to 250–300 mg every 8 hours. Generally, it is recommended that dosage increases be made no more often than every third day. Dosage should be decreased in the presence of hepatic insufficiency.

Electrophysiologic effects

Moricizine does not display the same affinity for the sodium channel displayed by other Class IC drugs. Hence, its effect on conduction velocity is less pronounced than that for flecainide or propafenone. In addition, moricizine decreases the action potential duration and therefore decreases refractory periods, similar to Class IB agents. Classification of moricizine has thus been controversial; some classify it as a Class IB drug. It is classified as a Class IC drug in this book mainly to emphasize its proarrhythmic effects (which are only rarely seen with Class IB drugs).

Hemodynamic effects

Moricizine may have a mild negative inotropic effect, but in general, exacerbation of congestive heart failure has been uncommon with this drug.

Therapeutic uses

Moricizine is moderately effective in the treatment of both atrial and ventricular arrhythmias. It has been used successfully in treating bypass-tract-mediated tachyarrhythmias and may have some efficacy against atrial fibrillation and atrial flutter. Its efficacy against ventricular arrhythmias is generally greater than that of Class IB agents but is clearly less than that for other Class IC drugs. A tendency for higher mortality with moricizine compared with that for placebo was seen in CAST, but the study was terminated before the tendency reached statistical significance.

Adverse effects and interactions

In general, moricizine is fairly well tolerated. Most side effects are related to the gastrointestinal or central nervous systems, similar to Class IB drugs. Dizziness, headache, and nausea are the most common side effects.

Proarrhythmia clearly occurs with moricizine more often than it does with Class IB drugs but less often than that with other Class IC drugs.

Cimetidine increases moricizine levels and moricizine decreases theophylline levels.

Reference

1 Echt DS, Liebson PR, Mitchell B, et al. Mortality and morbidity in patients receiving encainide, flecainide or placebo. N Engl J Med 1991;324:781.

CHAPTER 4

Class II antiarrhythmic drugs; beta-blocking agents

Beta-blocking drugs exert antiarrhythmic effects by blunting the arrhythmogenic actions of catecholamines. Compared with other antiarrhythmic drugs, these agents are only mediocre at suppressing overt cardiac arrhythmias. Nonetheless, beta blockers exert a powerful protective effect in certain clinical conditions—they are among the few drugs that have been shown to significantly reduce the incidence of sudden death in any subset of patients (an effect they most likely achieve by helping to prevent cardiac arrhythmias).

Because of the success of the drugs in treating a myriad of medical problems, more than two dozen beta blockers have been synthesized and more than a dozen are available for clinical use in the United States. In contrast to Class I antiarrhythmic drugs, the antiarrhythmic effects of the various Class II drugs tend to be quite similar to one another.

Electrophysiologic effects of beta blockers

For practical purposes, the electrophysiologic effects of beta blockers are manifested solely by their blunting of the actions of catecholamines. The effect of beta blockers on the cardiac electrical system, then, reflects the distribution of adrenergic innervation of the heart. In areas where there is rich adrenergic innervation, beta blockers can have a pronounced effect. In areas where adrenergic innervation is sparse, the electrophysiologic effect of beta blockers is relatively minimal.

Since the sympathetic innervation of the heart is greatest in the sinoatrial (SA) and atrioventricular (AV) nodes, it is in these structures that beta blockers have their greatest electrophysiologic effects. In both the SA and AV nodes, phase 4 depolarization is blunted by beta-blocking agents, leading to a decrease in automaticity, and hence to a slowing in the heart rate. In the AV node, beta blockers cause a marked slowing in conduction and a prolongation in refractory periods. The drugs have relatively little effect on SA nodal conduction in normal individuals but can markedly prolong SA nodal conduction (leading to sinus nodal exit block and hence bradyarrhythmias) in patients with intrinsic SA nodal disease. Beta blockers have very little effect on conduction velocity or refractoriness in normal atrial or ventricular myocardium.

Beta blockers can have a profound electrophysiologic effect, however, in ischemic or damaged myocardium. By helping to prevent ischemia, the drugs can reduce the incidence of arrhythmias. Further, beta blockers raise the threshold for ventricular fibrillation in ischemic myocardium and have been shown to reduce the risk of ventricular fibrillation during ischemia. There is also evidence that beta blockers can help prevent the formation of reentrant arrhythmias in myocardium that has been damaged by ischemia. In such damaged myocardium, a maldistribution of autonomic innervation can arise and lead to regional differences in adrenergic stimulation. Regional differences can serve as substrate for reentrant tachyarrhythmias by creating localized differences in refractory periods. By "smoothing out" localized differences in autonomic stimulation, beta blockers may help to prevent arrhythmias.

Beta-blocking agents in the treatment of arrhythmias

Supraventricular arrhythmias

The major electrophysiologic effects of beta blockers are manifested in the SA and AV nodes; it should not be surprising that the efficacy of beta blockers in treating supraventricular arrhythmias is mainly related to the extent to which the arrhythmias depend on the SA and AV nodes. Beta blockers are most effective in treating those supraventricular arrhythmias in which the SA or AV nodes are included within the reentrant pathways (namely, SA nodal reentrant tachycardia, AV nodal reentrant tachycardia, and macroreentrant tachycardias associated with bypass tracts). In these cases, beta blockers can have a direct suppressive effect on the pathways of reentry; thus, they can often terminate the arrhythmias and can help prevent their recurrence.

For arrhythmias arising within the atrial muscle (automatic or reentrant atrial tachycardias, atrial fibrillation, and atrial flutter),

Table 4.1 Potential effects of beta-blocking drugs on supraventricular tachyarrhythmias

Terminate or prevent
AV nodal reentrant tachycardia
SA nodal reentrant tachycardia
Macroreentrant (bypass-tract-mediated) tachycardia
Slow ventricular response
Atrial tachycardia (automatic or reentrant)
Atrial fibrillation
Atrial flutter

beta blockers have only a minimal direct suppressive effect. In these atrial arrhythmias, however, beta blockers can still be quite useful in helping to control the ventricular response by increasing the refractory period of the AV node, and thus allowing fewer impulses to be transmitted to the ventricles. In rare patients, beta blockers also help to prevent arrhythmias arising in the atria. In such instances, the atrial arrhythmias appear to be catechol dependent and patients often relate the onset of their arrhythmias to exercise. The effects of beta blockers on supraventricular arrhythmias are summarized in Table 4.1.

Ventricular arrhythmias

In general, beta blockers are not particularly effective in suppressing ambient ventricular ectopy or ventricular tachycardias. In some circumstances, however, generally when arrhythmias are dependent on catecholamines or related to myocardial ischemia, beta blockers can be useful. Beta blockers are the drugs of choice, for instance, for exercise-induced ventricular arrhythmias. Beta blockers have also been shown to reduce the number of episodes of ventricular fibrillation during acute myocardial infarction, to significantly improve overall survival, and to reduce the risk of sudden death and recurrent infarction in survivors of myocardial infarction.

Beta blockers can also be effective in treating some types of congenital long QT-interval syndrome. These syndromes are characterized by long QT intervals and a propensity for syncope or sudden death during exercise or during times of severe emotional stress. While the arrhythmias associated with these conditions are probably mediated by delayed afterdepolarizations, they are also apparently associated with localized differences in refractory periods caused by a maldistribution of sympathetic fibers in the ventricles. Beta blockers, which along with left stellate sympathectomy have been effective in treating many patients with these disorders, can help to smooth out any resultant sympathetic imbalance, reduce nonuniform refractory periods, and make arrhythmias less likely.

Clinical pharmacology of beta-blocking agents

To a large extent, all the available beta blockers appear to be of comparable efficacy in the treatment of arrhythmias and ischemia. Choosing among these agents for the purpose of treating arrhythmias is, then, mainly a matter of selecting a drug with an appropriate pharmacologic profile for the patient being treated. Among the considerations in making such a selection are the relative potencies of the drugs being considered and whether they offer receptor selectivity, intrinsic sympathomimetic activity (ISA), vasodilator activity, and membrane-stabilizing activity. Table 4.2 is not all inclusive, but it lists the pharmacologic properties of the most commonly used beta-blocking agents.

Potency of a beta blocker is not a major consideration, but the recommended dosages of various beta blockers differ markedly, and dosages must be adjusted accordingly for the drug being used.

Receptor selectivity refers to β_1-receptors (those in the heart) and β_2-receptors (those in the peripheral vasculature and bronchi). Drugs with selectivity, such as atenolol and metoprolol, produce minimal blockade of β_2-receptors and thus are potentially safer to

Table 4.2 Clinical pharmacology of beta-blocking drugs

Drug	β_1-Selective	ISA	Class I	Vasodilator	Lipid soluble	Half-life (h)
Acebutolol	+	+	+	0	Moderate	3–10
Atenolol	++	0	0	0	Weak	6–9
Carvedilol	0	0	++	+	Moderate	7–10
Esmolol	++	0	0	+	Weak	9 min
Labetolol	0	+	0	+	Weak	3–4
Metoprolol	++	0	0	0	Moderate	3–4
Pindolol	0	++	+	0	Moderate	3–4
Propranolol	0	0	++	0	High	3–4
Timolol	0	0	0	0	Weak	4–5

ISA, intrinsic sympathomimetic activity.

use in patients with lung disease or with impaired peripheral circulation.

ISA refers to the fact that some beta blockers, such as pindolol and acebutolol, produce a partial agonist (stimulating) effect on the beta receptor sites to which they bind (and block). Thus, in theory, heart rate depression and depression of myocardial function might not be as potent with beta blockers offering ISA. However, clear-cut clinical indications for using ISA drugs have not been identified. Of note, drugs offering ISA may not have a protective effect in survivors of myocardial infarction.

Vasodilator activity is produced by some beta blockers either through alpha-receptor blockade (carvedilol), or direct β_2-receptor stimulation (dilevalol), or both (labetolol).

Membrane-stabilizing activity refers to the fact that a few beta blockers exhibit Class I antiarrhythmic activity (slowing of the depolarization phase of the action potential) if serum levels are sufficiently high. However, the blood levels that must be achieved to demonstrate such Class I activity are greatly in excess of therapeutic levels. Thus, whether membrane-stabilizing activity is ever relevant with the use of beta blockers is very questionable.

The lipid solubility of beta blockers partially determines how the agents are metabolized (lipid-soluble drugs are generally metabolized in the liver and water-soluble drugs are generally excreted by the kidneys) and whether they cross the blood–brain barrier (drugs that cross are more prone to cause central nervous system side effects, such as fatigue, depression, insomnia, or hallucinations).

In summary, beta blockers as a class generally exhibit similar degrees of effectiveness in the treatment of cardiac arrhythmias. The major considerations in choosing among these drugs are the predominant route of elimination (to avoid accumulation of the drug in a patient with liver or kidney disease), side effects, and whether receptor selectivity or vasodilation are desired. In general, the potential for membrane-stabilizing activity should be ignored and ISA avoided.

Adverse effects and drug interactions

The most common side effects of beta blockers are a direct consequence of adrenergic blockade. These include bronchoconstriction, claudication, Raynaud's phenomenon, intensification of hypoglycemic episodes, and fatigue. Notably, while blocking sympathetic stimulation to the heart can lead to some degree of myocardial depression, patients with heart failure only rarely deteriorate significantly after the careful addition of beta blockers. In fact, beta blockers improve survival in patients with heart failure. Bradycardia due to adrenergic blockade is a well-recognized side effect of beta blockers, but patients only rarely develop symptomatic bradyarrhythmias on these drugs unless they have underlying SA nodal or AV nodal disease.

The sudden withdrawal of beta blockers, especially the short-acting beta blockers like propranolol, can lead to unstable ischemic heart disease in patients with underlying coronary artery disease. The withdrawal syndrome is substantially less likely with the longer-acting beta blockers.

Other possible but much less common side effects of beta blockers include rashes, fever, sexual dysfunction, mental depression, and gastrointestinal symptoms. In diabetics, beta blockers can mask symptoms of hypoglycemia and can cause hypoglycemia by reducing gluconeogenesis or hyperglycemia by reducing insulin levels.

Some of the side effects related to beta blockade itself may be avoided by appropriate drug selection. As noted, drugs with β_2-selectivity might help in avoiding bronchospasm, worsening of hypoglycemia, claudication, and Raynaud's phenomenon in some individuals. Using drugs with low lipid solubility might help to prevent central nervous system side effects.

Hepatic metabolism of lipid-soluble beta blockers can be increased by cimetidine and decreased by barbiturates. Aluminum hydroxide can delay absorption of beta blockers. The hepatic metabolism of lidocaine can be reduced by administration of lipophilic beta blockers, such as propranolol.

CHAPTER 5

Class III antiarrhythmic drugs

Class III antiarrhythmic drugs prolong the duration of the cardiac action potential, usually by blocking the potassium channels that mediate repolarization, and thus increase the refractory periods of cardiac tissue (Figure 5.1).

Despite this defining similarity, none of the currently available Class III drugs behave exactly alike. One reason the drugs are clinically dissimilar is that none are pure Class III agents—all have additional electrophysiologic effects that contribute to their efficacy and to their toxicity. Another reason for differences among the Class III drugs is that they display varying degrees of reverse use dependence.

The term *use dependence*, you may recall, refers to the time-related effect of Class I drugs on the sodium channel; as a result of binding kinetics, the degree of sodium-channel blockade increases as the heart rate increases. As it turns out, the magnitude of potassium-channel blockade manifested by Class III agents also is related to heart rate. For Class III drugs, however, the strength of blockade *decreases* as the heart rate increases; hence, the term *reverse use dependence* has been coined. Reverse use dependence means that at slower heart rates, the prolongation of the action potential is most pronounced; at faster heart rates, the effect diminishes. Reverse use dependence is related to a drug's binding characteristics. Drugs that preferentially bind to closed potassium channels, for instance, display significant reverse use dependence because phase 4 of the action potential is longer (and thus potassium channels spend more time in the closed state) when the heart rate is slow. Reverse use dependence has two potential undesirable effects. First, it causes some Class III drugs to lose potency with rapid heart rates, just when their potency is needed most. Second, the fact that action potential prolongation by some Class III drugs is most pronounced during bradycardia potentiates the tendency of these drugs to cause the pause-dependent early

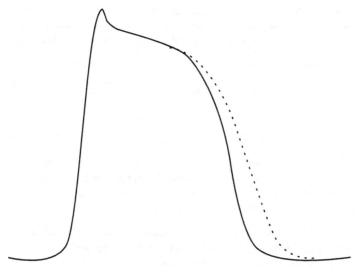

Figure 5.1 Effect of Class III drugs on cardiac action potential. Baseline action potential is displayed as a solid line; the dashed line indicates the effect of Class III drugs.

afterdepolarizations that produce torsades de pointes. Amiodarone is a unique Class III agent in several ways, as we will see, but one way it is different from other Class III drugs is that it binds preferentially to *open* potassium channels and therefore displays much less reverse use dependence. Consequently, amiodarone does not lose its effect when heart rate increases. The low magnitude of reverse use dependence seen with amiodarone may explain not only its remarkable efficacy against tachyarrhythmias but also its low incidence of producing torsades de pointes.

Although the differences among Class III drugs have not yet mandated that this class be formally subgrouped as the Class I drugs have been, it is necessary to keep in mind that these drugs are not interchangeable. The major clinical features of Class III antiarrhythmic drugs are listed in Table 5.1, and the major electrophysiologic properties are listed in Table 5.2.

Amiodarone

Amiodarone was synthesized in Belgium in the 1960s as a vasodilator, mainly for the purpose of treating angina. Its antiarrhythmic

Table 5.1 Clinical pharmacology of Class III drugs

	Amiodarone	Sotalol	Ibutilide	Dofetilide
GI absorption	30–50%	>90%	—	100%
Elimination	Hepatic*	Renal	Renal	Renal, some hepatic
Half-life	30–106 days	12 h	2–12 h	8–10 h
Dosage range	800–1600 mg/day for 3–10 days, then 100–400 mg/day PO	160–320 mg/day PO	10-mg IV infusion during 10 min, may be repeated	125–500 μg twice per day

*Both hepatic and renal elimination are minimal for amiodarone.
GI, gastrointestinal; IV, intravenous; PO, oral.

efficacy was noted in the early 1970s, and the drug rapidly came into widespread use in many European countries as an antiarrhythmic agent. In the late 1970s, clinical trials with amiodarone were begun in the United States and the oral form of the drug was approved by the Food and Drug Administration (FDA) in the mid-1980s. The intravenous form was approved in 1995.

Electrophysiologic effects

Amiodarone displays activity from all four antiarrhythmic classes. It is classified as a Class III antiarrhythmic drug because its major electrophysiologic effect is a homogeneous prolongation of the action potential, and therefore of refractory periods, due to blockade of the potassium channels. The drug has this Class III effect in all cardiac tissues. When therapy with amiodarone is first initiated, prolongation of refractoriness is not seen immediately. Instead, refractory periods gradually increase during the prolonged loading period (see below). Consequently, amiodarone's Class III drug effects may not become maximal for several weeks and notably, are not seen acutely even with intravenous loading of the drug.

In addition to its potassium-channel effects, amiodarone produces a mild-to-moderate blockade of the sodium channel (a Class I effect), a noncompetitive beta blockade (a Class II effect), and some degree

Table 5.2 Electrophysiologic properties of Class III drugs

	Amiodarone	Sotalol	Ibutilide	Dofetilide
Conduction velocity	Decrease +	0	0	0
Refractory periods	Increase ++	Increase ++	Increase ++	Increase ++
Automaticity	Suppress ++	Suppress +	Suppress +	Suppress +
Afterdepolarizations	May cause EADs	May cause EADs	May cause EADs	May cause EADs
Other effects	Class II and Class IV	Class II	None	None
Efficacy				
Atrial fibrillation/ atrial flutter	++	++	++	++
AVN reentry	+++	++	0	0
Macroreentry	+++	++	0	0
PVCs	+++	++	0	0
VT/VF	+++	++	0	+

AVN, AV node; EADs, early afterdepolarizations; PVCs, premature ventricular complexes; VT/VF, ventricular tachycardia and ventricular fibrillation.

of calcium-channel blockade (a Class IV effect). All these effects can produce antiarrhythmic actions.

Clinical pharmacology

The clinical pharmacology of amiodarone can be fairly described as being bizarre, complex, and incompletely understood. After an oral dose, 30–50% is absorbed from the gastrointestinal tract. Once absorbed, amiodarone displays a complex pattern of distribution that is usually described as (at least) a three-compartment model. The first, or central, compartment is thought to consist of the intravascular space. With aggressive loading regimens, the central compartment can be largely saturated within 24 hours. The second, or peripheral, compartment probably consists of most of the body's organs. It is thought to take 5–7 days to begin to saturate the peripheral compartment by use of a typical regimen for loading amiodarone— an important consideration because the antiarrhythmic effects of amiodarone are thought to require adequate filling of this peripheral compartment. The third, or deep, compartment consists of the body's fat. It takes many weeks or months for the third compartment to become saturated, and it may never actually become completely saturated. Because of the depth of this deep compartment, amiodarone has a huge volume of distribution, many times the body's actual volume; it has been calculated to be as high as 500 L. Tissue concentrations of amiodarone vary markedly from organ to organ and are the highest in organs with high-fat content, such as the liver and the lungs. In vivo, amiodarone is in a state of equilibrium among the three compartments. If the drug is discontinued, the concentration of amiodarone in the central compartment (the serum) falls quickly to low levels, but the low serum levels persist for weeks or months because of the slow leaching of the drug from the peripheral and deep compartments.

Amiodarone is metabolized in the liver to desethylamiodarone (DEA), which displays electrophysiologic effects similar to the parent compound and has similar pharmacologic properties. Very little amiodarone or DEA is excreted in the urine or the stool; essentially, amiodarone is stored, not excreted. Its chief means of elimination may actually be the gradual and natural sloughing of amiodarone-packed epithelial cells. The half-life of the drug has been reported as being between 2 weeks and 3 months in duration. This extraordinarily long half-life is reflected in the low daily dosage requirement after loading has been achieved.

Dosage

The unusual kinetics of amiodarone dictate the loading schedule. Usually, 1200–1600 mg/day are given orally in divided doses for several days (usually, 5–14 days), followed by 400–600 mg/day for several weeks, and finally by a chronic maintenance dose of 200–400 mg/day. This sort of loading regimen was derived empirically, but it is a logical approach. By giving large doses for days to weeks, one can achieve relatively rapid saturation of the central and peripheral compartments. Achieving a steady state, however, requires filling the deep compartment, which takes many weeks.

When treating non-life-threatening arrhythmias or when using amiodarone as prophylaxis against arrhythmias that are not manifest, a much gentler loading regimen is often used. Less aggressive loading schedules may avoid some toxicities associated with administering higher doses of the drug but require significantly more time to achieve both an antiarrhythmic effect and a steady state.

The use of intravenous amiodarone is generally reserved for the treatment of recurrent life-threatening ventricular tachyarrhythmias that have not responded to other therapies. The Class III effects of amiodarone are not seen acutely with IV loading; relatively long-term administration of the drug is necessary before prolongation of refractoriness is seen, just as with oral loading. The immediate effects of intravenous amiodarone are limited mainly to its Class II (beta-blocking) actions (Table 5.3), though some Class I effect (sodium-channel blockade) is also seen acutely. Accordingly, the most prominent electrophysiologic effect is prolongation of the

Table 5.3 Electrophysiologic effects of IV versus PO amiodarone*

Administration	QT interval	AH interval	Atrial RP	Ventricular RP
PO	Increase	Increase	Increase	Increase
IV	—	Increase	—	—

*The AH interval reflects the refractory period of the AV node. PO administration of amiodarone (after sufficient loading) results in prolongation of the action potential, as reflected by the resultant increase in the QT interval and in atrial and ventricular refractory periods; acute IV loading does not. The Class III effects of amiodarone are not seen with acute IV loading; instead, the increase in AV nodal refractoriness indicates that the Class II (and possibly Class IV) effects of amiodarone predominate.

RP, refractory periods.

atrioventricular (AV) nodal refractory periods, and the most prominent hemodynamic effect is hypotension. Any immediate antiarrhythmic efficacy with intravenous amiodarone is likely to be at least partially related to how dependent a patient's arrhythmias are on catecholamine stimulation. When amiodarone is loaded intravenously, 1 g is delivered during the first 24 hours as follows: 150 mg is infused during the first 10 minutes (15 mg/min), followed by 360 mg during the next 6 hours (1 mg/min), and then followed by 540 mg during the next 18 hours (0.5 mg/min). If intravenous therapy is still desired after the first 24 hours, the infusion can continue at 0.5 mg/min (720 mg/24 h).

Indications

Amiodarone is a broad-spectrum antiarrhythmic agent. It can be efficacious for virtually any type of tachyarrhythmia, though it is approved by the FDA only for the treatment of ventricular tachyarrhythmias.

Amiodarone is the most effective drug yet developed for recurrent ventricular fibrillation or hemodynamically unstable ventricular tachycardia. Early studies with amiodarone generally limited its use to patients whose ventricular tachyarrhythmias had proven refractory (most often, as documented during electrophysiologic testing) to other antiarrhythmic therapy. Even in this difficult-to-treat population, amiodarone reduced the risk of sudden death to about half that seen with more conventional drugs. In subsequent randomized trials, however, amiodarone proved to be significantly inferior to the implantable defibrillator in reducing mortality. The main indications for oral amiodarone today in the treatment of ventricular arrhythmias are to either reduce the frequency of shocks in patients who have implantable defibrillators or offer at least partially effective therapy to patients deemed not to be candidates for an implantable defibrillator.

Amiodarone is moderately effective in maintaining sinus rhythm in patients with atrial tachyarrhythmias, including atrial fibrillation and atrial flutter. In patients with heart failure, amiodarone is probably the drug of choice after cardioversion for atrial fibrillation, since it has few adverse hemodynamic effects, and often results in a well-controlled ventricular response should the arrhythmia recur. (The use of antiarrhythmic drugs in the treatment of atrial fibrillation will be discussed in Chapter 11.) Amiodarone is also effective in bypass-tract-mediated tachycardias and AV nodal reentrant tachycardias.

However, these arrhythmias can almost always be cured with ablation procedures, and amiodarone should be used very rarely in their management.

Adverse effects and interactions

Amiodarone causes a high incidence of side effects, ranging from merely annoying to life threatening. Many side effects of amiodarone appear to be related to the total lifetime cumulative dose of the drug (rather than to the daily dosage). Even when low daily dosages are used, therefore, significant side effects are seen, and the risk of developing new side effects continues to increase as therapy continues over time. Side effects occur in approximately 15% of patients during the first year but increase to over 50% with chronic therapy. Adverse effects require discontinuation of the drug in approximately 20% of patients. It has been widely speculated that much of the unique organ toxicity seen with amiodarone is related to the iodine atoms contained in the drug, a feature not shared by any other antiarrhythmic drug.

Gastrointestinal side effects are common but, in most cases, are relatively mild. Nausea, vomiting, or anorexia have an incidence of approximately 25% during the high-dose loading phase, but these symptoms often improve with lowering of the daily dosage. Esophageal reflux caused by an amiodarone-induced paralysis of the lower esophageal sphincter is an uncommon but potentially devastating side effect.

Elevation of hepatic transaminases of up to twice normal values is seen in about 25% of patients treated with amiodarone. In most cases, these elevations return toward normal after a few months, although amiodarone-induced hepatitis has been reported in approximately 3% of patients. When hepatic transaminases remain chronically elevated, the consequences are unclear. Occasional cases of cirrhosis have been reported, however.

Pulmonary complications are generally considered the most dangerous side effect seen with amiodarone and are the form of toxicity most likely to prove fatal. Acute adult respiratory distress syndrome from amiodarone-induced pneumonitis can be seen at any time during therapy, but the time of highest risk is probably immediately after surgery, especially cardiac surgery. The incidence of acute amiodarone-induced pneumonitis is generally reported to be 2–5%, but the cumulative incidence may be higher with long-term therapy. A chronic interstitial fibrosis can also be seen with amiodarone; the incidence of this problem is unclear. The carbon monoxide (CO) diffusing capacity is almost always depressed with amiodarone-induced pulmonary problems, but this laboratory finding is unfortunately nonspecific—many patients taking amiodarone develop depressed CO diffusing capacities without clinically apparent pulmonary problems. Therefore, routine pulmonary function tests do not appear to help in predicting which patients will eventually develop lung toxicity.

Thyroid problems with amiodarone are relatively common. Amiodarone reduces peripheral conversion of T4–T3, resulting in somewhat increased T4 levels and somewhat decreased T3 levels even in euthyroid patients. Approximately 10% of patients treated with amiodarone eventually develop true hypothyroidism (a low serum T4 level is always significant in patients taking this drug), and a smaller proportion develop hyperthyroidism. Although hypothyroidism can be treated relatively easily with thyroid-replacement medication, hyperthyroidism represents a difficult clinical problem because of its presentation and its treatment. Amiodarone-induced hyperthyroidism sometimes manifests as an exacerbation of the patient's underlying ventricular tachyarrhythmias. This is a potentially lethal condition. Further, because amiodarone itself contains a significant amount of iodine, patients receiving amiodarone have high-iodine stores, which thus precludes the use of radioactive iodine for thyroid ablation. To make matters worse, treating amiodarone-induced hyperthyroidism with antithyroid drugs can be difficult or even impossible. Sometimes thyroidectomy is the only feasible means of controlling amiodarone-induced hyperthyroidism.

Cutaneous side effects with amiodarone are relatively frequent. Significant photosensitivity occurs in about 20% of patients taking the drug, and some patients eventually develop a blue-gray discoloration of sun-exposed skin, which can be quite disfiguring.

Neurologic side effects are rare but can include ataxia, tremor, sleep disturbances, and peripheral neuropathy. A proximal myopathy can also be seen with amiodarone.

Ocular symptoms (most often, poor night vision or halo vision) occasionally accompany the corneal microdeposits seen in virtually all patients taking amiodarone.

Multiple drug interactions have been reported with amiodarone. The most common are the potentiation of warfarin and increased digoxin levels. Quinidine, procainamide, phenytoin, and flecainide levels are also increased. As a rule, if amiodarone is given in combination with Class I antiarrhythmic drugs, the dosage of the Class I drug should be decreased. Amiodarone can potentiate the effect of beta blockers and calcium blockers and lead to negative inotropic effects and bradyarrhythmias.

Sotalol

Sotalol, a noncardioselective beta blocker, was initially developed as an antihypertensive agent. Its Class III antiarrhythmic properties were noted in 1970, and it began to be studied as an antiarrhythmic agent at that time. It was approved by the FDA for the treatment of ventricular arrhythmias in 1993 and is now also approved for the treatment of atrial fibrillation.

Electrophysiologic properties

Sotalol is a Class III antiarrhythmic drug; it produces prolongation of the cardiac action potential in both the atria and the ventricles. It produces a dose-related prolongation in the QT interval, which appears to reflect both its antiarrhythmic properties and its propensity to cause torsades de pointes. It is actually a racemic mixture of D-sotalol (which has Class III effects) and L-sotalol (which has both Class III effects and beta-blocking effects). As a beta blocker, sotalol is about one-third as potent as propranolol. Sotalol displays reverse use dependence, so its effect—including QT-interval prolongation—increases with lower heart rates.

Clinical pharmacology

Sotalol is well absorbed from the gastrointestinal tract, and peak plasma concentrations occur within 2–3 hours after an oral dose. The drug is not metabolized; it is excreted unchanged by the kidneys, and the dosage should be reduced in patients with renal insufficiency. The elimination half-life is 7–8 hours.

Dosage

The usual starting dosage of sotalol is 80 mg twice daily, and the dosage is increased gradually, as needed, to 240–320 mg/day in divided doses. Intervals of at least 2 or 3 days between dosage increments are recommended. Careful monitoring of the QT interval must be performed while titrating the dose because the risk of developing torsades de pointes with sotalol is clearly related to QT-interval prolongation. The corrected QT interval should be kept below 500 milliseconds to keep the risk of torsades de pointes under 2%. Dosage greater than 320 mg/day may be necessary to suppress arrhythmias, but higher doses lead to a substantial increase in the incidence of torsades de pointes (as high as 11% in patients whose corrected QT interval exceeds 550 ms).

Indications
Sotalol is approved for the treatment of significant ventricular arrhythmias but can be useful for treating all types of tachyarrhythmias. The drug is generally considered more effective than Class IA drugs but not as effective as amiodarone.

Adverse effects and drug interactions
The major side effects of sotalol are related to its noncardioselective beta-blocking effects (e.g., bradyarrhythmias, negative inotropy, and exacerbation of asthma) and to its propensity to cause torsades de pointes. Exacerbation of congestive heart failure is most commonly seen in patients whose left ventricular ejection fractions are less than 0.35, especially if the patients also have a history of heart failure.

Torsades de pointes is of more concern with sotalol than it is with Class IA drugs or with amiodarone. As noted, the risk of torsades de pointes with sotalol is directly related to the magnitude of its Class III effects, as reflected by the duration of the QT interval. The higher the dose and the longer the QT interval, the higher the risk. Because sotalol displays reverse use dependence, its effect on the QT interval is even more profound at slower heart rates. So, for instance, if sotalol is being used to treat atrial fibrillation, the relative safety of using the drug (i.e., the magnitude of QT-interval prolongation) must be assessed during sinus rhythm, that is, when the heart rate is slowest and the risk of torsades de pointes is highest. Thus, such a patient should never be sent home taking sotalol until he or she has been observed in sinus rhythm. Hypokalemia also magnifies the incidence of sotalol-induced torsades de pointes. Therefore, the drug should be used with trepidation in patients taking potassium-wasting diuretics—another good reason to avoid the drug in patients with congestive heart failure. A multicenter randomized trial using D-sotalol in patients with ventricular arrhythmias was stopped because of an excess of sudden death in the D-sotalol arm. Presumably, torsades de pointes was largely responsible for the excess mortality.

Concomitant use of Class IA drugs can greatly magnify the risk of torsades de pointes. Sotalol can potentiate, in an additive fashion, the negative inotropic and bradyarrhythmic effects of other beta-blocking agents and of calcium-blocking drugs.

Ibutilide

Ibutilide is a newer Class III antiarrhythmic agent, approved by the FDA in its intravenous form for the acute cardioversion of atrial fibrillation and atrial flutter.

Electrophysiologic properties
Ibutilide is a unique Class III drug in that it causes prolongation of the action potential by blocking inward sodium currents in addition to outward potassium currents. Like sotalol, the drug produces a dose-related prolongation in the QT interval and displays reverse use dependency.

Clinical pharmacology
After intravenous infusion, ibutilide is extensively metabolized to eight metabolites. More than 80% of the drug is excreted in the urine, only 7% as unmetabolized ibutilide. The elimination half-life is variable (2–12 h) but averages 6 hours. The drug is subject to pronounced first-pass metabolism when given orally, which is why only the intravenous form is available.

Dosage
Ibutilide is infused as a 1-mg intravenous bolus during a period of 10 minutes. If the arrhythmia being treated (atrial fibrillation or atrial flutter) persists for 10 minutes after the infusion has been completed, a second 1-mg bolus can be administered. The infusion should be stopped immediately if the target arrhythmia is terminated or if ventricular arrhythmias or a marked prolongation of the QT interval is seen. After the infusion has been completed, the patient should be observed on a cardiac monitor for at least 4 hours or until the QT interval returns to normal, whichever is longer.

Indications
Ibutilide is indicated for the elective conversion of atrial fibrillation or atrial flutter. It should be thought of as an alternative to elective direct-current (DC) cardioversion. In clinical studies, the efficacy of ibutilide administration in terminating these arrhythmias (after two 1-mg doses) was 44%.

Adverse effects and drug interactions

The major adverse effect of ibutilide is its propensity to cause torsades de pointes. During clinical trials, ibutilide was not given to patients whose corrected QT intervals were greater than 440 milliseconds, and serum potassium levels were required to be greater than 4.0 mEq/L. Despite these precautions, ventricular tachyarrhythmias were seen in some patients. Sustained ventricular arrhythmias requiring emergent cardioversion were seen in 1.7%, and nonsustained ventricular tachycardias were seen in 4.9%. The incidence of sustained ventricular arrhythmias was much higher in patients with a history of congestive heart failure (5.4%). Most ventricular arrhythmias were seen within 1 hour of the drug infusion, but some were seen nearly 3 hours after the infusion. It is thought that the arrhythmogenic potential of ibutilide is increased when it is used with other drugs that prolong the duration of the action potential. Thus, ibutilide should not be used with Class IA or other Class III antiarrhythmic drugs, nor should these drugs be administered within 4–6 hours after infusion of ibutilide. Ibutilide should also be avoided in patients receiving phenothiazines, tricyclic antidepressants, tetracyclic antidepressants, or antihistamine agents that block the H_1 receptor.

Clinical utility of ibutilide

The overall clinical utility of ibutilide probably ought to be considered marginal, mainly because of the disadvantages of the drug. Since only approximately 40% of patients are effectively treated with ibutilide, more than half of the patients treated with the drug still will require DC cardioversion. The incidence of torsades de pointes with ibutilide is also troubling, and the relatively prolonged monitoring required after its use (regardless of whether it is effective) can be quite inconvenient.

Dofetilide

Dofetilide is a Class III antiarrhythmic drug, approved by the FDA in 1999 for the treatment of atrial fibrillation. Significant restrictions were placed on its usage, however.

Electrophysiologic properties

Dofetilide is considered a "pure" Class III drug in that it blocks a single potassium channel resulting in prolongation of the action potential and of refractory periods in both the atria and the ventricles, but—in contrast to amiodarone and sotalol—it does not have any other antiarrhythmic properties. Like other Class III drugs, it displays a dose-dependent prolongation of the QT interval and reverse use dependence (so QT-interval prolongation is more pronounced at lower heart rates). Its major side effect, typical for drugs with these electrophysiologic properties, is torsades de pointes.

Clinical pharmacology

Dofetilide is fully absorbed after oral administration. While it is eliminated by both the kidneys and the liver, the renal route of elimination is particularly important clinically. The dosage of the drug needs to be carefully adjusted in patients with reduced creatinine clearances. In healthy patients, the elimination half-life is 8–10 hours.

While the measurement of blood levels of dofetilide is not available clinically, there is a very close correlation between plasma concentration and the QT interval. Careful measurements of the QT interval, therefore, are used to titrate dosage.

Clinical use

When the FDA approved dofetilide, it significantly restricted its usage. The drug is available only to hospitals and physicians that have been certified to administer it and is dispensed only by a limited number of pharmacies. Certification is achieved by completing an educational program provided by Pfizer, the manufacturer.

Patients must be hospitalized to receive dofetilide. First, a corrected QT interval and a creatinine clearance are obtained; if the QTc is above 440 milliseconds or the creatinine clearance is below 20 mL/min, the drug cannot be used. The initial dose is adjusted for the creatinine clearance. If the creatinine clearance is greater than 60 mL/min, 500 μg of dofetilide is given twice a day. If the creatinine clearance is between 40 and 60 mL/min, 250 μg twice a day is given. If the creatinine clearance is between 20 and 40 mL/min, 125 μg twice a day is given.

Between 2 and 3 hours after the first dose of dofetilide is given, the QTc is recalculated. If the increase in the QTc is less than or equal to 15%, the initial dosage is continued. If the increase in QTc is 15% or higher, or if the QTc is greater than 500 milliseconds, the dosage is reduced. If, at any time after the second dose, the QTc is above 500 milliseconds, dofetilide should be discontinued.

Continuous, in-hospital monitoring is required for at least 72 hours and at least 12 hours after conversion to sinus rhythm.

Indications

Dofetilide is indicated for conversion to normal sinus rhythm, and especially for the maintenance of sinus rhythm, in patients with atrial fibrillation or atrial flutter. Because of the drug's narrow therapeutic to toxic ratio, and the extraordinary precautions that must be taken in using it, dofetilide is generally reserved for patients whose arrhythmias are highly symptomatic.

Dofetilide is moderately effective in converting atrial fibrillation and atrial flutter to sinus rhythm. With doses of 500 μg, conversion within 24–36 hours has been reported to occur in 30–70% of patients.

Dofetilide appears to be more useful in maintaining sinus rhythm after successful conversion. If dosages of 500 μg twice per day can be maintained, 60–65% of patients treated with dofetilide have been reported to remain in sinus rhythm for up to 12 months after conversion from atrial fibrillation. Doses less than 500 μg twice per day were much less effective in clinical trials, but these doses were chosen by randomization and not by titrating according to renal function and QT intervals.

Only very limited information is available on the efficacy of dofetilide for ventricular arrhythmias. The drug is not approved for this indication.

Adverse effects and drug interactions

By far, the most important adverse effect of dofetilide is torsades de pointes, the bane of Class III antiarrhythmic drugs. Torsades de pointes was seen in as few as 1% but as many as >3% of patients given dofetilide in clinical trials. Reducing the odds of experiencing this arrhythmia requires careful titration of the drug, and reducing death from torsades de pointes requires prolonged in-hospital monitoring. The need to take such precautions has led to an extraordinarily restrictive approval status for dofetilide in the United States.

Dofetilide has minimal hemodynamic effects and can be used in patients with heart failure.

Dofetilide has been reported to cause occasional noncardiac symptoms, including headache, gastrointestinal disturbances, sleep disorders, and flulike symptoms.

Drug interactions are very important with dofetilide. Dofetilide is completely contraindicated with drugs that can reduce its elimination and thus increase its plasma concentration. These drugs include verapamil, cimetidine, trimethoprim, prochlorperazine, and megestrol. It should also be avoided in combination with drugs that can also prolong the QT interval, including all Class I and Class III antiarrhythmic drugs, tricyclic antidepressants, erythromycin, phenothiazines, cisapride, bepridil, and, in fact, any of the other drugs listed in Table 1.3. It should be used with caution with triamterene, metformin, and amiloride, which are drugs that compete with dofetilide for priority in the renal transport system.

CHAPTER 6
Class IV drugs: calcium-blocking agents

Of the many calcium-blocking agents that have been developed, only two are commonly used (and have been approved) for the treatment of cardiac arrhythmias: verapamil and diltiazem. For many other calcium-blocking agents, such as nifedipine, vasodilatory effects predominate; for these agents, reflex responses to vasodilation appear to counteract and cancel any cardiac electrophysiologic effects. Therefore, this chapter is limited to a discussion of verapamil and diltiazem.

Clinical pharmacology of verapamil and diltiazem

When verapamil is given orally, more than 90% is absorbed, but first-pass hepatic metabolism reduces bioavailability to 20–35%. Approximately 90% of the drug is protein bound. With chronic administration, the elimination half-life is 5–12 hours. Very little verapamil is excreted unchanged in the urine. Verapamil can be given as an intravenous bolus for the emergent termination of reentrant supraventricular arrhythmias.

Diltiazem, like verapamil, is well absorbed but is also subject to first-pass metabolism, yielding a bioavailability of about 40%. Diltiazem is 70–80% protein bound. The drug is metabolized in the liver, and the elimination half-life is approximately 3.5 hours. Diltiazem is also available for intravenous infusion and is occasionally used in this form to control heart rate during atrial fibrillation or atrial flutter.

Dosage
The usual dosage of verapamil is 240–360 mg/day in divided doses given every 8 hours. Diltiazem is given four times a day, with a usual dosage range of 180–360 mg/day. Both drugs are also available in long-acting forms that can be given once or twice a day.

Verapamil can be given intravenously as a bolus. Five to 10 mg is administered over a period of 2 minutes; an additional 10 mg can be given after 10 minutes. When giving diltiazem intravenously, 0.25 mg/kg (approximately 20–25 mg) should be given as a bolus over a period of 2 minutes, followed by infusion at 10 mg/h. Infusion rates can be titrated to as much as 15 mg/h, depending on the response of the heart rate. Continuing diltiazem infusions for longer than 24 hours is not recommended because longer infusion periods have not been studied.

Electrophysiologic effects of calcium-blocking agents

Calcium-blocking agents inhibit the slow calcium channel that is responsible for the depolarization of the sinoatrial (SA) and atrioventricular (AV) nodes. Accordingly, the major electrophysiologic effects of calcium-channel blockers are limited to these two structures. Both verapamil and diltiazem depress automaticity, slow conduction, and increase refractoriness in both the SA and AV nodes. The drugs, therefore, are particularly useful in arrhythmias utilizing the AV node as part of the reentrant circuit.

As a general rule, calcium blockers have minimal or no electrophysiologic effect on the atrial or ventricular myocardium. However, the slow calcium channel has been invoked as a necessary component in the development of both early afterdepolarizations and delayed afterdepolarizations. Accordingly, calcium-channel blockers can occasionally ameliorate afterdepolarizations and the arrhythmias they cause.

Further, it is apparent that the calcium channels might be responsible, on occasion, for localized areas of slow conduction in the ventricles. Thus, in relatively rare circumstances, calcium-channel blockers can be used to treat ventricular arrhythmias (see below, and Chapter 12)

Like Class I antiarrhythmic drugs, calcium blockers exhibit use dependence—their binding and blocking of the calcium channels increases at more rapid heart rates.

Clinical use of calcium-blocking agents

Supraventricular tachyarrhythmias

Verapamil and diltiazem can be very useful in the management of many supraventricular tachyarrhythmias either by affecting the

mechanism of the arrhythmia itself and thus terminating or preventing it, or in slowing the ventricular response to the arrhythmia.

Atrial tachyarrhythmias

All these arrhythmias are localized to the atrial myocardium, so calcium blockers have very little direct effect on them. However, because calcium blockers increase the refractory period of the AV node,
they can be very helpful in controlling the ventricular response during atrial tachyarrhythmias.

In general, it is easier to control ventricular response during
atrial fibrillation than it is during atrial flutter or atrial tachycardia. With the latter two arrhythmias, changes in the ventricular
rate response do not occur smoothly, as they most often do in atrial
fibrillation; instead, they occur in discrete "jumps," changing suddenly, for instance from 2:1 AV conduction to 3:1 or 4:1 conduction.
This sort of quantum response tends to be difficult to achieve. On
the other hand, controlling the ventricular response during chronic
atrial fibrillation is often quite achievable, though a combination of
drugs may be required (calcium blockers plus beta blockers and/or
digoxin). In the acute setting, intravenous infusions of diltiazem
have proven to be very effective in controlling the ventricular rate
during atrial tachycardias.

Multifocal atrial tachycardia

Multifocal atrial tachycardia is almost exclusively seen during acute
illness, most often during acute respiratory decompensation. The
arrhythmia is currently thought to be mediated by afterdepolarizations. Accordingly, verapamil can sometimes improve the arrhythmia itself instead of merely increasing the degree of AV block.

AV nodal reentry and macroreentrant tachycardias

Reentrant arrhythmias that use the AV node as part of the reentrant circuit are very susceptible to therapy with calcium blockers.
Calcium blockers terminate these arrhythmias by slowing AV nodal
depolarization and increasing refractoriness. As a result of these electrophysiologic effects, *Mobitz I AV block* occurs (second-degree AV
block characterized by a progressive prolongation of AV nodal conduction before a nonconducted impulse). Since these arrhythmias
require conduction through the AV node, producing a single blocked
impulse in the AV node is sufficient to terminate them. Verapamil
by intravenous bolus is extremely effective (>90%) in terminating

these arrhythmias acutely. Both verapamil and diltiazem are moderately effective in preventing recurrences of these reentrant arrhythmias.

Ventricular tachyarrhythmias

As noted, the slow calcium channel has very little to do with depolarization of the typical myocardial cell. Accordingly, neither verapamil nor diltiazem are efficacious in treating typical reentrant ventricular tachyarrhythmias.

Two clinical syndromes have been described, however, in which verapamil has been effective in treating ventricular tachycardia—repetitive monomorphic ventricular tachycardia (which seems to be due to a channelopathy) and idiopathic left ventricular tachycardia (which may be a form of reentrant tachycardia involving abnormal, verapamil-sensitive Purkinje fibers). These syndromes are discussed in more detail in Chapter 12.

Toxicity and drug interactions

Verapamil has significant negative inotropic properties and can precipitate congestive heart failure in patients with impaired ventricular function. Like any calcium blocker (many of which are marketed solely for the treatment of hypertension), verapamil can produce significant hypotension. Other side effects include constipation, dizziness, nausea, headache, edema, and bradyarrhythmias. (These latter are seen almost exclusively in patients with underlying SA nodal or AV nodal conduction disease.) Hypotension can be additive when verapamil is used with other antihypertensive agents. Negative inotropic effects can be additive when verapamil is given with flecainide, disopyramide, or beta blockers. Verapamil can increase drug levels of carbamazepine , cyclosporine, and theophylline. Rifampin and phenobarbital can reduce levels of verapamil. Verapamil can reduce serum lithium levels in patients taking lithium; on the other hand, verapamil can increase sensitivity to lithium.

Diltiazem also has negative inotropic properties but clinically significant impairment of ventricular function caused by diltiazem has been rare. Similar to verapamil, diltiazem can produce bradyarrhythmias and hypotension. Elevations in hepatic transaminases have been reported. Other side effects include dermatitis, headache, dizziness, and weakness.

The side effects of bradycardia, hypotension, and possibly, deterioration of ventricular function can be additive when diltiazem is used with beta blockers or antihypertensive agents. Cimetidine and ranitidine can increase diltiazem levels. Diltiazem can increase levels of digoxin, cyclosporine, and carbamazepine.

CHAPTER 7

Unclassified antiarrhythmic agents

Digoxin, adenosine, and magnesium are often used to treat cardiac arrhythmias. Since these agents do not fit the Vaughan-Williams classification system (see Chapter 2), they are considered separately in this chapter.

Digoxin

Digitalis preparations have been used in clinical medicine since the 1700s. Digoxin, the preparation of digitalis now most commonly used, is well absorbed, is excreted by the kidneys, and has an elimination half-life of 1.7 days.

The clinical utility of digoxin is twofold. First, it increases intracellular calcium during muscle contraction, thus increasing inotropy. Second, it increases parasympathetic tone, which makes it useful for treating supraventricular arrhythmias.

Since parasympathetic innervation is greatest in the sinoatrial (SA) and atrioventricular (AV) nodes, they are the structures whose electrophysiology is most affected by digoxin. Thus, digoxin can be beneficial in any arrhythmia in which the AV node plays a critical role, such as AV nodal reentrant tachycardia (in which the AV node is a direct participant in the arrhythmia itself), and in atrial fibrillation and atrial flutter. In atrial fibrillation and atrial flutter, digitalis has little or no direct effect on the arrhythmia itself but can be useful in slowing the ventricular response by increasing the refractory period of the AV node. Digoxin can also be of benefit in treating bypass-tract-mediated tachycardias, but because the drug can have a direct effect on the bypass tract itself (resulting in a shortening of refractoriness and thus potentially making the bypass tract more dangerous), it is rarely used for these arrhythmias.

Digoxin is a well-tolerated drug, as long as toxic levels are avoided. Digitalis toxicity, however, can be a serious clinical problem

manifested by gastrointestinal symptoms (nausea, vomiting, anorexia, diarrhea, and cramps), neurologic symptoms (visual disturbances, restlessness, and delirium), and significant arrhythmias (SA
nodal dysfunction, AV block, atrial tachycardia, junctional tachycardia, and ventricular tachycardia). The cardiac arrhythmias associated
with digoxin toxicity are potentially life threatening. Digoxin toxicity appears to increase the risk of developing refractory ventricular
arrhythmias or bradyarrhythmias after direct-current cardioversion;
cardioversion should be avoided if digoxin levels are high. The manifestations of digoxin toxicity are exacerbated by hypokalemia, and
maintaining normal serum potassium levels in patients taking this
drug is important.

Management of digoxin toxicity consists of stopping the drug, cor-
recting electrolyte disturbances (especially, hypokalemia and hypomagnesemia), pacing (if significant bradyarrhythmias are present),
and using phenytoin or lidocaine for ventricular arrhythmias. If life-
threatening arrhythmias are present, use of digoxin-specific anti-
bodies can be rapidly effective and should be considered.

Digoxin levels can be elevated by concomitant use of quinidine,
amiodarone, verapamil, erythromycin, and tetracycline. Digoxin
levels can be lowered by cholestyramine and neomycin.

Adenosine

Adenosine is a naturally occurring nucleoside that, in high concentration, has a profound but fleeting depressive effect on the SA and
AV nodes. When given intravenously, the effect of adenosine is maximal after 10–30 seconds and is manifested by transient high-degree
AV block, profound slowing of the SA node, or both. Transient AV
block is the mechanism by which the drug terminates supraventricular tachyarrhythmias (Figure 7.1). The drug is removed from the
circulation very quickly; its half-life is less than 10 seconds. In addition to its electrophysiologic effects, adenosine can have a potent
vasodilatory effect, but this effect is also fleeting.

Adenosine has proven very useful for the acute termination
of reentrant tachyarrhythmias that involve the AV node. Almost
100% of AV nodal reentrant tachycardias and bypass-tract-mediated
macroreentry can be terminated by an intravenous bolus of adenosine. The drug is also helpful in diagnosing the mechanism of wide-
QRS complex tachycardia—it terminates AV nodal and macroreentrant arrhythmias; causes transient heart block, which transiently

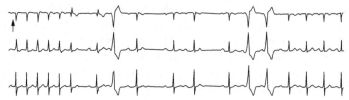

Figure 7.1 Termination of supraventricular tachycardia with adenosine. The figure illustrates termination of an episode of AV nodal reentrant tachycardia by administration of a bolus of intravenous adenosine. Surface ECG leads V1, II, and V5 are shown, top to bottom, respectively. Within seconds of administering adenosine (arrow), tachycardia abruptly terminates.

slows atrial tachyarrhythmias; and generally has no effect on ventricular tachycardia (Table 7.1).

The drug is given as a rapid intravenous bolus, usually beginning with 6 mg intravenously for 1–2 seconds. A 12-mg bolus can be used if no effect occurs within 2 minutes.

Adenosine often causes transient bradyarrhythmias. Flushing, headache, sweating, and dizziness are also relatively common, but these symptoms last for less than 1 minute. Rare cases of exacerbation of asthma have been reported with adenosine.

Magnesium

Magnesium has not received as much attention as other electrolytes, which reflects a general, recurrent theme and shortcoming in science—if something is difficult to measure, it tends to be ignored despite its potential importance. Not only is the metabolism of magnesium complicated (absorption from the gut is highly variable and depends on the level of magnesium in the diet, and the

Table 7.1 Effect of adenosine on various tachyarrhythmias

Termination	Transient slowing of heart rate	No response
SA nodal reentry	Atrial tachycardia	Ventricular tachycardia
AV nodal reentry	Atrial fibrillation	
Macroreentrant SVT	Atrial flutter	

SVT, supraventricular tachycardia.

renal excretion of magnesium is also difficult to study) but serum levels of magnesium only poorly reflect body stores. Thus, there is no simple test to assess the status of a patient's magnesium stores.

Recently, however, there has been growing interest in the use of intravenous magnesium to treat a variety of medical conditions (in addition to its traditional place in the treatment of preeclampsia): asthma, ischemic heart disease, and cardiac arrhythmias. The most well-established use for parenteral magnesium is treatment of arrhythmias.

The precise mechanism by which magnesium can ameliorate arrhythmias has not been established. That magnesium might have an effect on cardiac electrophysiology is not surprising, however, when one considers that among the many enzyme systems in which magnesium plays a crucial role is the sodium–potassium pump. Magnesium can thus have an important influence on sodium and potassium transport across the cell membrane and therefore on cardiac action potential.

The most well-established use of magnesium as an antiarrhythmic agent is in the therapy of torsades de pointes. Most likely, magnesium has a suppressive effect on the development of the afterdepolarizations responsible for this arrhythmia. Whatever the mechanism, because of its efficacy, rapidity of action, and relative safety, intravenous magnesium has become the drug of first choice in the acute treatment of torsades de pointes. Magnesium appears to be effective in this condition even when there is no evidence of magnesium depletion.

Magnesium may also have a role to play in treating arrhythmias associated with digitalis toxicity. The inhibition of the sodium–potassium pump mediated by digoxin (which may play a role in digitalis-toxic arrhythmias) appears to be countered by magnesium administration. Indeed, magnesium deficiency itself may play a role in the genesis of the arrhythmias because digoxin tends to cause magnesium wasting.

Because magnesium slows conduction in the AV node, some have reported terminating supraventricular tachyarrhythmias by giving intravenous magnesium. Although one would expect magnesium to be most effective in terminating arrhythmias in which the AV node plays a crucial role, there are a few reports suggesting that magnesium can sometimes also terminate multifocal atrial tachycardia. Magnesium administration may also help prevent postoperative arrhythmias after cardiac surgery.

Table 7.2 Symptoms of magnesium toxicity

Serum Mg ++ Levels (mEq/L)	Symptoms
5–10	ECG changes (increased PR interval and QRS duration)
10–15	Loss of reflexes
15–20	Respiratory paralysis
20–25	Cardiac arrest

ECG, electrocardiogram.

Whether magnesium deficiency is a prerequisite for benefit from the intravenous administration of magnesium is not clear. Still, magnesium deficiency can cause or exacerbate cardiac arrhythmias (and cause tremors, tetany, seizures, potassium depletion, and psychiatric disturbances), so it is important to take a patient's magnesium stores into account when treating arrhythmias. A low serum magnesium level often reflects low-magnesium stores, but low total magnesium may exist in the absence of hypomagnesemia. Thus, one needs to have a high index of suspicion for magnesium depletion. Especially if symptoms compatible with magnesium depletion are present, magnesium therapy should be considered in patients presenting with malnutrition, alcohol abuse, diabetes, hypokalemia, hypocalcemia, and in patients taking amphotericin B, cyclosporine, digoxin, gentamicin, loop diuretics, or pentamidine.

For the acute treatment of cardiac arrhythmias, the administration of intravenous magnesium has proven very safe. There is some potential of pushing magnesium levels into the toxic range in the presence of severe renal failure, but the overall risk of doing so is low. (Symptoms associated with toxic magnesium levels are listed in Table 7.2.) Eight to 16 mEq of magnesium (1–2-g magnesium sulfate) can be infused rapidly over several minutes. A total of 32 mEq (4 g) can be given during 1 hour if necessary. Oral therapy is inappropriate for the acute treatment of cardiac arrhythmias because of the variable (and limited) absorption of magnesium from the gastrointestinal tract. Chronic oral administration of magnesium salts may be helpful in some conditions, such as in patients receiving loop diuretics.

CHAPTER 8
Investigational antiarrhythmic drugs

This chapter offers brief descriptions of some of the more promising investigational antiarrhythmic drugs likely to become available for clinical use over the next few years. The task of developing new drugs and bringing them to market is fraught with risk, and with antiarrhythmic drugs, this risk may be even higher than usual. It is entirely possible that any of the following four drugs might fall by the wayside before they gain final approval for clinical use.

Azimilide

Azimilide (Proctor & Gamble) is a Class III antiarrhythmic agent that is being evaluated for the treatment of both supraventricular and ventricular tachyarrhythmias. Azimilide displays at least two unique and potentially beneficial electrophysiologic properties.

First, while all Class III drugs block the potassium channels responsible for repolarization, and thus extend the duration of the action potential, azimilide causes a unique form of potassium-channel blockade. The inward potassium current that mediates repolarization can be resolved into two separate components—the rapidly activating current, or I_{Kr}; and the slowly activating current, or I_{Ks}. Typical Class III agents, including sotalol, ibutilide, and dofetilide, block only the I_{Kr} current. Azimilide, on the other hand, blocks both components of the inward potassium current. It has been postulated that the imbalanced blockade of the potassium current produced by typical Class III drugs contributes to the development of afterdepolarizations, and thus to the development of torsades de points. The more "balanced" blockade offered by azimilide, in theory, may reduce the risk of this type of proarrhythmia.

Second, while typical Class III agents display reverse use dependence, in which their potassium-channel-binding increases at slower heart rates and decreases at faster heart rates, azimilide does not. Instead, its potassium-channel-blocking effect is independent of heart rate. In general, reverse use dependence is a detriment to the effectiveness of antiarrhythmic drugs. Because these drugs are intended to treat tachyarrhythmias, it is generally not a useful thing for them to lose efficacy at faster heart rates. Furthermore, because drugs displaying reverse use dependence produce greater potassium-channel blockade at slower heart rates, these drugs are more likely to produce torsades de pointes at these slower (i.e., nontachyarrhythmic) heart rates.

Thus, both the balanced potassium-channel blockade and the lack of reverse use dependence displayed by azimilide offer the promise that the risk of torsades de pointes may be lower with this drug than for other Class III agents.

Azimilide produces a dose-dependent prolongation in the QT interval, and little or no hemodynamic effect. In early clinical trials, the most frequently reported side effect is headache. A potentially very troublesome problem, however, is that rare cases of early neutropenia (within 6 weeks of initiation) have been reported, which, at this time, appears to reverse when the drug is stopped.

Several clinical trials with azimilide have been conducted to date testing the drug in the treatment of supraventricular arrhythmias, and several additional trials are ongoing. Its efficacy in the prevention of recurrent atrial fibrillation appears to be similar to that of other Class III drugs. At this point, while the risk of torsades de pointes appears to be lower than that for other Class III drugs (less than 1%), this problem clearly has not been completely eliminated with azimilide.

Interestingly, azimilide is also being evaluated for the treatment of ventricular arrhythmias. New drugs aimed at ventricular arrhythmias have become a rarity in recent years, since the widespread adoption of the implantable defibrillator and the recognition that antiarrhythmic drugs (aside from amiodarone) often increase mortality in patients with underlying heart disease. In the randomized Azimilide Postinfarct Survival Evaluation (ALIVE) trial [1], azimilide was compared to placebo as primary prophylaxis in nearly 4000 myocardial infarction survivors with reduced ejection fractions. There was no difference in the 1-year overall mortality in the two groups.

However, the incidence of new onset atrial fibrillation was significantly reduced in the group receiving azimilide.

While it is probably disappointing to the manufacturers of azimilide that this drug did not reduce mortality when used as primary prophylaxis in high-risk patients, it is noteworthy that (unlike virtually every other antiarrhythmic agent except amiodarone) it did not *increase* mortality in these patients. An additional trial is ongoing to examine the utility of azimilide in reducing recurrent ventricular tachyarrhythmias in patients with implantable defibrillators. Having an effective agent to use in this clinical situation, in addition to amiodarone, would be quite helpful.

Thus, azimilide is a unique investigational Class III antiarrhythmic agent whose efficacy against supraventricular arrhythmias appears to be on a par with other Class III drugs, whose efficacy against ventricular arrhythmias is at least promising, and whose propensity to cause torsades de pointes may be less than for some other Class III drugs.

Dronedarone

If one were to ask electrophysiologists to describe the ideal antiarrhythmic drug, most would probably describe a drug that was as effective as amiodarone but without its incredible array of toxicities. Indeed, an "amiodarone without the side effects" is virtually the Holy Grail of antiarrhythmic drugs. Dronedarone (developed by Sanofi-Aventis, also the developer of amiodarone) is a derivative of amiodarone and is held by some to potentially be that Holy Grail.

The dronedarone molecule is a modified version of amiodarone. The major difference is that dronedarone lacks the iodine atoms that are a major feature of amiodarone. The iodine in amiodarone is almost certainly responsible for its thyroid toxicity, so it is a good bet that dronedarone will not cause similar thyroid-related side effects. Furthermore, the lack of iodine in dronedarone makes the drug significantly less lipophilic than amiodarone, and much of the organ toxicity of amiodarone is speculated to be due to its affinity for fat.

Dronedarone, like its cousin, is a multichannel blocker. It displays not only Class III properties but also fairly prominent Class I properties, as well as some Class IV (calcium-blocking) properties. Like amiodarone, acute administration of dronedarone does not appear to produce any Class III effects—instead, its acute effects are related to its sodium-channel-blocking activity. Class III effects are seen after 2–3 weeks of use. Initial clinical trials have been promising. In over 1200 patients presenting with atrial fibrillation or atrial flutter, dronedarone proved significantly more effective than placebo in preventing recurrence of the atrial arrhythmias. Additionally, dronedarone appears to be useful in controlling the ventricular response in patients with chronic atrial fibrillation when therapy with digitalis, beta blockers, and calcium blockers has failed. Often, such patients are referred for atrioventricular nodal ablation and placement of a permanent pacemaker. A pharmacologic solution to rate control in these patients would obviously be an attractive alternative to ablating the patient into a state of permanent complete heart block.

From available evidence, however, the efficacy of dronedarone in preventing the recurrence of atrial tachyarrhythmias is not obviously more striking than for other nonamiodarone Class III antiarrhythmic drugs. Head-to-head trials will be necessary to prove any exceptional antiarrhythmic efficacy.

The toxicity profile of dronedarone to this point appears quite favorable. In clinical trials to date, none of the thyroid, lung, or hepatic toxicity so prominent with amiodarone has been seen. Furthermore, neither torsades de pointes nor other forms of proarrhythmia have been seen.

Overall, whether or not dronedarone proves to be the Holy Grail thus far it does appear to be a very promising addition to the arsenal of antiarrhythmic drugs.

Tedisamil

Tedisamil (Solvay Pharmaceuticals) is a Class III antiarrhythmic drug being developed for the treatment of atrial fibrillation and atrial flutter.

Tedisamil, like all Class III drugs, blocks potassium channels and thus prolongs the action potential duration. It is not nearly a "pure" Class III drug, however, since it blocks several other channels as well. In the atria, it blocks at least one of the channels responsible for phase 4 depolarization, an effect that tends to produce bradycardia. The bradycardic effect of tedisamil, in fact, led to its initially being evaluated as an antianginal agent.

An early clinical trial with tedisamil showed that it effectively converted atrial fibrillation of recent onset when given intravenously.

Unfortunately, the drug also produced torsades de pointes in some patients. Because of a relatively high incidence of apparent proarrhythmia, the clinical program with tedisamil has been temporarily suspended. While the manufacturer hopes to develop tedisamil as both an intravenous agent for acute conversion of atrial fibrillation and an oral agent for maintaining sinus rhythm, the status of the drug at this writing is questionable.

Piboserod

Piboserod (Bio-Medisinsk Innovasjon, BMI) is a prospective antiarrhythmic drug that does not fit any of the Vaughan-Williams drug classes. Piboserod is a 5-HT4 receptor antagonist; that is, it blocks serotonin.

5-HT4 receptors are present in the human atrium, and when stimulated, they cause increased chronotropic and inotropic effects on atrial tissue. Not surprisingly, therefore, it has been asserted that serotonin can induce atrial tachyarrhythmias. Piboserod, which blocks serotonin receptors in the atria, is being evaluated as a drug that might suppress atrial fibrillation. Piboserod is also being evaluated in the treatment of heart failure and irritable bowel syndrome.

Reference

1 Camm AJ, Pratt CM, Schwartz PJ, et al. Mortality in patients after a recent myocardial infarction. A randomized, placebo-controlled trial of azimilide using heart rate variability for risk stratification. Circulation 2004;109:990–996.

CHAPTER 9
Common adverse events with antiarrhythmic drugs

The decision to use an antiarrhythmic drug always exposes the patient to at least some risk of an adverse outcome. This chapter considers in detail three varieties of adverse events that are common to many antiarrhythmic drugs: proarrhythmia, drug–drug interactions, and drug–device interactions.

Proarrhythmia

It may seem paradoxical that drugs designed to suppress cardiac arrhythmias may instead worsen them or even produce arrhythmias that did not initially exist. Proarrhythmia begins to make sense, however, when one considers that most arrhythmias ultimately are caused by some change in the cardiac action potential and that most antiarrhythmic drugs work by causing changes in the cardiac action potential. We always hope that the changes in the action potential produced by an antiarrhythmic drug will make arrhythmias less likely to occur. However, whenever we choose to use these drugs, we must accept the possibility that the opposite might happen.

At least four categories of drug-induced proarrhythmia can be seen: bradyarrhythmias, worsening of reentry, torsades de pointes, and arrhythmias resulting from worsening hemodynamics.

Bradyarrhythmias

Antiarrhythmic drugs can abnormally slow the heart rate by suppressing the sinoatrial (SA) node or by causing atrioventricular (AV) block. Generally speaking, however, only patients who already have underlying disease in the SA node, AV node, or His-Purkinje system are likely to experience symptomatic slowing of the heart rate with antiarrhythmic drugs.

Sinus bradycardia can be seen with any drug that suppresses the SA node—beta blockers, calcium blockers, or digitalis. Again, however, symptomatic sinus slowing is almost never seen in patients who do not have some degree of intrinsic SA nodal dysfunction. The most common example of a symptomatic, drug-induced sinus bradyarrhythmia (and probably the most common cause of syncope in patients with SA nodal dysfunction) is the prolonged asystolic pause that can be seen when a drug is used to convert atrial fibrillation. The phenomenon occurs because diseased SA nodes display exaggerated overdrive suppression. Overdrive suppression is the phenomenon, seen even in normal SA nodes, whereby several seconds of atrial tachycardia temporarily suppresses SA nodal automaticity. As a result, when the atrial tachycardia suddenly stops, the SA node fires at a relatively slow rate for several cardiac cycles. In diseased SA nodes, this transient "slowing" of intrinsic automaticity can become exaggerated and prolonged. In these cases, the addition of an antiarrhythmic drug might even further suppress SA nodal automaticity, resulting in prolonged episodes of asystole when an atrial tachyarrhythmia abruptly terminates. Unfortunately, SA nodal disease is relatively common in patients with atrial tachyarrhythmias because the two disorders are often part of the same disease process—both the propensity to atrial tachyarrhythmias and the SA nodal dysfunction are caused by diffuse fibrotic changes in the atria. AV nodal block can occur when beta blockers, calcium blockers, digoxin, or any combination of these drugs are used in patients with underlying AV nodal disease. Digitalis toxicity is the most common cause of drug-induced AV nodal block.

Class IA, Class IC, or occasionally Class III drugs can produce block in the His-Purkinje system in patients who have underlying distal conducting system disease. Because subsidiary pacemakers distal to the His bundle are unreliable when distal heart block occurs, antiarrhythmic drugs should be used with particular care in patients with known or suspected distal conducting system disease.

In general, the treatment of drug-induced bradyarrhythmias is to discontinue the offending agent and use temporary or permanent pacemakers as necessary to maintain adequate heart rate.

Worsening of reentrant arrhythmias

Figure 9.1 reviews how antiarrhythmic drugs can work to benefit reentrant arrhythmias. By changing the conduction velocity, refractoriness, or both in various parts of the reentrant circuit,

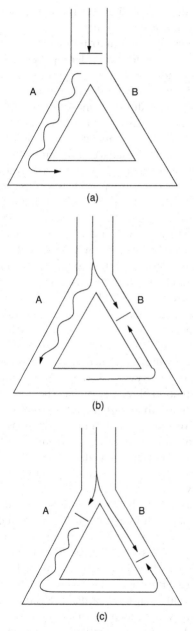

Figure 9.1 Effect of antiarrhythmic drugs on a reentrant circuit (same as Figure 2.3).

antiarrhythmic drugs can eliminate the critical relationships necessary to initiate and sustain reentry.

Chapter 2 discussed how antiarrhythmic drugs can worsen reentrant arrhythmias. To review, consider a patient who has an occult reentrant circuit whose electrophysiologic properties do not support a reentrant arrhythmia. Giving the patient mexiletine, a drug that reduces action potential duration, may preferentially reduce the refractory period of one pathway, giving this circuit the characteristics shown in Figure 9.1a, and thus making a reentrant arrhythmia much more likely to occur. A similar scenario can be developed for a patient with the circuit shown in Figure 9.1c and who is given sotalol, a drug that prolongs refractory periods (see also Figure 2.3).

Unfortunately, whenever an antiarrhythmic drug is given to a patient with a potential reentrant circuit, the drug may render an arrhythmia less likely to occur or it may render an arrhythmia more likely to occur. This sad truth follows because the mechanism that produces an antiarrhythmic effect (namely, the alteration of conduction velocity and refractory periods) is the very same mechanism that produces a proarrhythmic effect.

Exacerbation of reentrant tachycardias can occur whether one is treating supraventricular or ventricular arrhythmias. The risk of producing this type of proarrhythmia is highest with Class IC drugs (since profound slowing of conduction velocity is a particularly good way to potentiate reentry), but it is also fairly common with Class IA drugs. Exacerbation of reentry can also be seen with Class IB and Class III drugs, but with less frequency. Class II and Class IV drugs rarely produce worsening of reentrant arrhythmias and usually only in patients with supraventricular arrhythmias that utilize the AV node as part of the reentrant circuit.

Clinically, this form of proarrhythmia is manifested by an increase in the frequency or duration of a reentrant arrhythmia. Not uncommonly, and especially with Class IC drugs, a reentrant arrhythmia that had occurred only infrequently will suddenly become relatively incessant. Since the drugs most commonly producing this sort of proarrhythmia (i.e., Class IA and Class IC drugs) cause a slowing in conduction velocity, often the proarrhythmic tachycardia occurs at a slower rate than did the original tachycardia. If the arrhythmia being exacerbated is ventricular tachycardia, the clinical manifestation of proarrhythmia may be sudden death.

Treating any drug-related exacerbation of a reentrant arrhythmia requires the recognition that the "new" arrhythmia is caused by a drug. This recognition, in turn, requires a high index of suspicion. In general, one should be alert for any sign of proarrhythmia whenever treating a reentrant arrhythmia with antiarrhythmic drugs. If proarrhythmia is suspected, the offending drugs should be immediately stopped and the patient supported hemodynamically until the drug metabolizes (a particular problem when using a drug with a long half-life). Proarrhythmic reentry, like spontaneous reentry, can often be terminated by antitachycardia pacing techniques. If needed, a temporary pacemaker can be placed for antitachycardia pacing until the patient stabilizes. Adding additional antiarrhythmic drugs when this type of proarrhythmia is present often only makes things worse and should be avoided if possible.

Torsades de pointes

Torsades de pointes is the name given to the polymorphic ventricular tachycardias associated with prolonged QT intervals or other repolarization abnormalities. As outlined in Chapter 1, these arrhythmias are thought to be caused by the development of afterdepolarizations, which, in turn, are a common result of using antiarrhythmic drugs.

Drugs that increase the duration of the cardiac action potential—Class IA and Class III drugs—can produce the pause-dependent ventricular tachyarrhythmias that are mediated by early afterdepolarizations. As shown in Chapter 1 (see Figure 1.16), the arrhythmias generally present as frequent, recurrent bursts of polymorphic ventricular tachycardia preceded by a pause. They are often relatively asymptomatic, but they can also produce syncope or death.

Proarrhythmia caused by this mechanism should be strongly suspected whenever a patient being treated with quinidine, procainamide, disopyramide, sotalol, or dofetilide complains of episodes of light-headedness or syncope. In the case of sotalol and dofetilide, the risk of torsades de pointes is directly related to the degree of QT-interval prolongation—the longer the QT interval, the higher the risk. Such a direct association with the QT interval is much less clear with Class IA drugs. The incidence of torsades de pointes with most Class IA and Class III drugs is generally estimated to be at least 2–5%.

Toxic levels of digoxin can produce polymorphic ventricular tachycardia by causing delayed afterdepolarizations (see Figure 1.15b). This type of arrhythmia is not pause dependent. A new onset of polymorphic ventricular tachycardia or the development of syncope in patients treated with digoxin should prompt measurement of a digoxin level.

Worsening of hemodynamics

Much less well documented are the arrhythmias that occur as a result of drug-induced cardiac decompensation or hypotension. Acute cardiac failure can lead directly to arrhythmias by causing abnormal automaticity (i.e., the so-called intensive care unit arrhythmias). Hypotension can cause arrhythmias by the same mechanism or by causing reflex sympathetic stimulation. Thus, antiarrhythmic drugs that decrease the inotropic state of the heart (beta blockers, calcium blockers, disopyramide, or flecainide) or drugs that cause vasodilation (calcium blockers, some beta blockers, and the intravenous administration of quinidine, procainamide, bretylium, or amiodarone) can occasionally lead to cardiac arrhythmias.

Proarrhythmia in perspective

Although the potential for antiarrhythmic drugs to worsen cardiac arrhythmias has been known for decades, the potential magnitude of the problem has been recognized for only a few years. The single most important event that drew attention to the problem of proarrhythmia was the reporting of the results of the Cardiac Arrhythmia Suppression Trial (CAST) [1]. In CAST, survivors of myocardial infarction who had reduced left ventricular ejection fractions and complex ventricular ectopy were randomized to placebo or to one of three Class IC antiarrhythmic drugs (encainide, flecainide, or moricizine) that had been shown previously to suppress their ectopy. The hypothesis of the study was that suppressing these patients' ambient ectopy would improve their mortality. Instead, the results showed that patients treated with encainide or flecainide had a fourfold increase in the risk of sudden death (patients treated with moricizine showed no benefit from drug treatment) and had a significant increase in overall mortality. The increase in risk for fatal arrhythmias was not limited to the first few days or weeks of drug therapy but persisted throughout the follow-up period.

CAST proved to be a major blow to the Class IC drugs in particular, but evidence suggests that its results might also apply, at least to some extent, to other antiarrhythmic agents. Other trials have suggested, for instance, that uses of both quinidine for atrial fibrillation and Class I drugs in survivors of myocardial infarction have produced significant increases in mortality.

As a result, most electrophysiologists have become convinced that the proarrhythmic effects of Class I drugs outweigh the antiarrhythmic effects, at least in patients with underlying heart disease. Lately,

Table 9.1 Relative risk of drug-induced proarrhythmia

Drug	Risk of exacerbation of reentry	Risk of torsades de pointes
Class IA		
Quinidine	++	++
Procainamide	++	++
Disopyramide	++	++
Class IB		
Lidocaine	+	0
Mexiletine	+	0
Phenytoin	+	0
Class IC		
Flecainide	+++	0
Propafenone	+++	0
Moricizine	+++	+
Class III		
Amiodarone	+	+
Sotalol	+	+++
Ibutilide	+	+++
Dofetilide	+	+++

it has been fashionable in some circles to extol the relative virtues of Class III drugs, but with the likely exception of amiodarone, these drugs too carry a significant risk of proarrhythmia. Using antiarrhythmic drugs always involves the risk of making heart rhythm worse instead of better. (For each drug, the relative risks of causing the major forms of proarrhythmia are shown in Table 9.1). One should prescribe these drugs only if it is necessary for prolongation of survival or for amelioration of significant symptoms. Most importantly, whenever one is compelled to prescribe antiarrhythmic drugs, one should feel obligated to do whatever possible to minimize the risk of symptomatic or life-threatening proarrhythmia.

Since reentrant ventricular tachycardia (and therefore drug-induced worsening of reentry) generally is seen only in the presence of underlying cardiac disease, one must be especially cautious about using antiarrhythmic drugs in patients with heart disease. When prescribing antiarrhythmic drugs in this setting, it is important to assure that serum electrolytes (especially potassium) are kept well within the normal range. In addition, cardiac function should be optimized because hemodynamic compromise can worsen arrhythmias. Cardiac ischemia should be managed aggressively. Not only does ischemia itself precipitate arrhythmias, but ischemia also renders drug-induced proarrhythmia more likely.

Torsades de pointes probably occurs in individuals who are genetically prone to develop afterdepolarizations whenever their cardiac action potentials become prolonged. Thus, underlying heart disease is not necessary for this form of proarrhythmia—any patient treated with a Class IA or Class III drug is a potential candidate for torsades de pointes (at least until practical genetic screening for torsades de pointes becomes available). Patients started on therapy with such drugs should be placed on a cardiac monitor for several days, because torsades de pointes is most often first seen during the initial 3 or 4 days of therapy (although it can occur any time). With sotalol and dofetilide, the QT interval should be monitored carefully during drug loading. Serum potassium levels should also be watched carefully; in fact, one should use torsades de pointes producing agents with trepidation in patients requiring potassium-wasting diuretics.

Drug–drug interactions

Antiarrhythmic drugs seem to produce more than their share of interactions with other drugs. Interactions generally are related to competition with other drugs for serum proteins on which to bind or to drug-induced changes in hepatic metabolism. The major interactions between antiarrhythmic drugs and other agents (see the discussions of the individual antiarrhythmic drugs) are summarized in Table 9.2.

Drug–device interactions

Antiarrhythmic drugs can occasionally interfere with the function of electronic pacemakers and implantable cardioverter defibrillators (ICDs). It is relatively rare for antiarrhythmic drugs to significantly interfere with pacemakers. Class IA drugs can increase pacing thresholds, but only at toxic drug levels. Class IC drugs, sotalol, and amiodarone can increase pacing thresholds at therapeutic levels, but only rarely to a clinically important extent. The effects of antiarrhythmic drugs on pacing thresholds are summarized in Table 9.3. The interaction of antiarrhythmic drugs with ICDs can occur in

Table 9.2 Major drug interactions of antiarrhythmic drugs

Drug	Levels increased	Levels decreased	Levels or effect increased	Levels or effect decreased
Class IA				
Quinidine	Amiodarone	Phenobarbital Phenytoin Rifampin	Anticholinergics Warfarin Phenothiazines Digoxin	
Procainamide	Amiodarone Trimethoprim Cimetidine	Ethanol		
Disopyramide		Phenobarbital Phenytoin Rifampin		
Class III				
Lidocaine	Propranolol Metoprolol Cimetidine	Phenobarbital		
Mexiletine	Cimetidine Choramphenicol Isoniazid	Phenytoin Phenobarbital Rifampin	Theophylline Lidocaine Phenytoin	

(Continued)

Table 9.2 (*Continued*)

Drug	Levels increased	Levels decreased	Levels or effect increased	Levels or effect decreased
Phenytoin	Cimetidine Isoniazid Sulfonamides Amiodarone	Theophylline	Theophylline Quinidine Disopyramide Lidocaine Mexiletine	
Class IC Flecainide	Amiodarone Cimetidine Propranolol Quinidine		Digoxin	
Propafenone	Cimetidine Quinidine	Phenobarbital Phenytoin Rifampin	Digoxin Propranolol Metoprolol Theophylline Cyclosporine Desipramine Warfarin	

Moricizine	Cimetidine	Theophylline
Class III		
Amiodarone	Warfarin	
	Digoxin	
	Class I drugs	
	Beta blockers	
	Calcium blockers	
Sotalol	Class IA drugs*	
	Beta blockers	
Ibutilide	Class IA drugs*	

*Produce additive risk of torsades de pointes.

Table 9.3 Effect of antiarrhythmic drugs on pacing thresholds

Increase at normal drug levels	Increase at toxic drug levels	No increase
Flecainide	Quinidine	Lidocaine
Propafenone	Procainamide	Mexiletine
Amiodarone	Disopyramide	
Sotalol		

several ways and is often clinically significant. Two major problems caused by antiarrhythmic drugs are that they can change the energy required for successful defibrillation and they can change the characteristics of the arrhythmia being treated.

The effect of antiarrhythmic drugs on defibrillation energy requirements is an important consideration because increasing the defibrillation threshold can render an ICD ineffective. The effects of various drugs on defibrillation energy requirements are summarized in Table 9.4. In general, drugs that block the sodium channel increase defibrillation energy requirements (thus, Class IC drugs have the most profound effect, and Class IA and Class IB drugs tend to have proportionally lesser effects), and drugs that block the potassium channels (e.g., sotalol) decrease defibrillation energy requirements. Drugs that affect both the sodium and potassium channels (i.e., Class IA drugs and amiodarone) have mixed effects—sometimes they increase and sometimes they decrease defibrillation energy requirements. If one must prescribe a drug that has the potential of increasing defibrillation energy requirements for a patient who has an ICD, one should consider retesting defibrillation thresholds after the drug has been loaded to be sure that the ICD is still capable of delivering sufficient energy to reliably defibrillate the patient.

Antiarrhythmic drugs can also interact with ICDs by changing the characteristics of a patient's ventricular tachycardia. By slowing the

Table 9.4 Effect of antiarrhythmic drugs on defibrillation thresholds

Increase	Mixed effect	Decrease
Flecainide	Quinidine	Sotalol
Propafenone	Procainamide	
Lidocaine	Amiodarone	
Mexiletine		

rate of ventricular tachycardia, a drug can render the arrhythmia more amenable to antitachycardia pacing, which potentially makes the ICD more effective. On the other hand, by slowing the rate of ventricular tachycardia below the recognition rate of the ICD, a drug can cause the ICD to fail to recognize (and therefore fail to treat) recurrent arrhythmias. Antiarrhythmic drugs can also cause reentrant ventricular arrhythmias to recur more frequently or even to become incessant, thus inducing frequent ICD therapy, which, in turn, can cause excessive discomfort and premature battery depletion of the ICD. In general, when one is compelled to add an antiarrhythmic drug to the treatment regimen of a patient with an ICD, one should consider electrophysiologic testing to reexamine the characteristics of the patient's arrhythmias and to be sure that the ICD is optimally programmed to treat the arrhythmias.

Reference

1 Echt DS, Liebson PR, Mitchell B, et al. Mortality and morbidity in patients receiving encainide, flecainide or placebo. N Engl J Med 1991;324:781.

Part 3

Antiarrhythmic drugs in the treatment of cardiac arrhythmias

CHAPTER 10

Basic principles of using antiarrhythmic drugs

The first two sections of the book concerned the mechanisms of cardiac arrhythmias, the mechanism of action of antiarrhythmic drugs, and the features of specific antiarrhythmic drugs. In this final section, that information is applied to the use of antiarrhythmic drugs in the treatment of specific cardiac arrhythmias. Chapter 10 reviews some basic principles that should be kept in mind when using antiarrhythmic drugs.

On the basis of the generally limited efficacy of antiarrhythmic drugs as well as their inherent propensity to cause serious problems, the first principle should be completely self-evident; namely, one should avoid using antiarrhythmic drugs whenever possible. Thus, when one has decided to prescribe an antiarrhythmic drug, the final step before actually writing the order should be to ask, "Does this patient really need this drug?" There are only two general conditions in which using an antiarrhythmic drug is entirely appropriate: first, when an arrhythmia needs to be suppressed because it threatens to cause death or permanent harm, and second, when an arrhythmia needs to be suppressed because it produces significant symptoms. Before prescribing an antiarrhythmic drug, the physician should be certain that the arrhythmia meets one of these two conditions.

The second basic principle is to keep the goal of treatment clearly in mind and to tailor the aggressiveness of one's therapy accordingly. If one is treating an arrhythmia to prevent death or permanent injury, for instance, a relatively aggressive approach may be appropriate and necessary. In theory, if the object is to spare life and limb, one should err on the side of efficacy, perhaps willingly accepting the risk of certain drug toxicities. In practice, however, as we will see in Chapters 11 and 12, there are relatively few instances today where one ought to rely primarily on antiarrhythmic drugs to treat arrhythmias that threaten life and limb.

On the other hand, if one is treating an arrhythmia to relieve symptoms, a more circumspect approach is appropriate. In these cases, one generally should use a stepwise strategy, beginning with milder, less risky forms of treatment, and carefully reassessing the risk-to-benefit ratio before each potential escalation of therapy. All too often physicians pursue the treatment of relatively insignificant arrhythmias with Ninja-like intensity, an error that can result in unnecessary injury or death.

The final basic principle of using antiarrhythmic drugs is that, if one feels compelled to expose a patient to the risk of the drugs, one should also feel compelled to take every reasonable precaution to reduce the risks. For instance, given the almost universal risk of proarrhythmia, one should often consider placing patients on a cardiac monitor while antiarrhythmic drugs are being initiated because, although proarrhythmia can occur any time during the course of treatment, a significant proportion of these events occur during the first 3 or 4 days of drug usage. Most importantly, one must take great care in deciding which drug to use. The choice must be individualized.

The accompanying tables summarize the factors that should be considered in choosing antiarrhythmic drugs for patients with and without significant underlying cardiac disease.

Some drugs are plainly contraindicated for particular patients. Procainamide, for instance, should not be used in patients with systemic lupus erythematosus; quinidine should not be used in patients with chronic colitis; patients with severe lung disease (in whom mild drug-induced pulmonary toxicity goes a long way) ideally should not receive amiodarone; patients with a history of heart failure should not receive drugs with negative inotropic effects.

Beyond these obvious individual considerations, the presence or absence of underlying heart disease is the most important variable in choosing an antiarrhythmic drug, because heart disease predisposes patients to reentrant circuits and, therefore, to proarrhythmia. As shown in Table 10.1, beta blockers and Class IB drugs are the safest choice regardless of whether the patient has underlying heart disease. Class IC drugs are reasonably safe for patients with normal hearts, but because they very frequently exacerbate reentrant ventricular tachyarrhythmias, they are to be avoided in patients with underlying cardiac disease. Class IA drugs carry a moderate risk of toxicity for patients without cardiac disease because they cause both torsades de pointes and end-organ toxicity; in patients with cardiac

Table 10.1 Relative overall risk of serious toxicity from antiarrhythmic drugs*

Increasing order of risk for patients with no underlying heart disease	Increasing order of risk for patients with underlying heart disease[†]
Class II	Class II
Class IB	Class IB
Class IC	Sotalol and dofetilide
Sotalol and dofetilide	Amiodarone
Class IA	Class IA
Amiodarone[‡]	Class IC (should not use)

*Ranking of relative risks takes into account the risk of both proarrhythmia and end-organ toxicity.

[†]For patients with underlying heart disease, the ranking changes because these patients have a much higher propensity for proarrhythmia. Amiodarone rises in rank because of its relatively low risk of producing proarrhythmia. Class IC drugs should virtually never be used in these patients.

[‡]For patients without underlying heart disease, its impressive range of end-organ toxicity makes amiodarone the riskiest drug.

disease, they also add a moderate risk of exacerbation of reentrant arrhythmias. Sotalol and dofetilide carry a moderate risk of torsades de pointes for all patients. Amiodarone carries a substantial risk of significant end-organ toxicity for all patients, though only a relatively small risk of proarrhythmia.

Table 10.2 ranks the efficacy of antiarrhythmic drugs for atrial and ventricular tachyarrhythmias and for atrioventricular (AV)-node-dependent arrhythmias. For atrial tachyarrhythmias, Class IA drugs, sotalol, and dofetilide, are roughly equal in efficacy. Class IC drugs and amiodarone are somewhat more effective than are Class IA drugs, and Class IB drugs have virtually no efficacy for these arrhythmias. Most antiarrhythmic agents have some degree of efficacy against AV-node-dependent arrhythmias. For ventricular tachyarrhythmias, Class II and Class IB drugs are least effective; amiodarone is most effective.

Table 10.3 synthesizes the data from Tables 10.1 and 10.2 to generalize about the potential drugs of choice for atrial and ventricular tachyarrhythmias (keeping in mind that drug selection must be individualized in every case). The main consideration is always to balance efficacy with safety.

Table 10.2 Increasing order of relative efficacy for tachyarrhythmias

Atrial tachyarrhythmias*	AV-node-dependent tachyarrhythmias†	Ventricular tachyarrhythmias
Class IA	Class IA	Class II
	Digoxin	Class IB
Sotalol	Class II	Class IA
Dofetilide	Verapamil‡	Class IC
Class IC	Sotalol	Sotalol
Amiodarone	Class IC	Amiodarone
	Amiodarone	
	Verapamil§	
	Adenosine	

*Atrial tachycardia, atrial fibrillation, and atrial flutter.
†AV-nodal reentry and macroreentry (bypass-tract-mediated).
‡When used orally for maintenance of sinus rhythm.
§When used intravenously for acute termination of the arrhythmia.

The drug of choice in treating both atrial and ventricular tachyarrhythmias depends on the presence or absence of underlying cardiac disease. For instance, in the absence of heart disease, Class IC drugs may offer the most favorable balance of efficacy and safety in the treatment of atrial tachyarrhythmias. However, in the presence of underlying heart disease, Class IC agents (because of their impressive propensity to exacerbate reentrant ventricular arrhythmias)

Table 10.3 Drugs of choice for atrial and ventricular arrhythmias*

Underlying heart disease absent		Underlying heart disease present	
Atrial arrhythmias†	Ventricular arrhythmias‡	Atrial arrhythmias	Ventricular arrhythmias
Class IC	Class II	Sotalol	Amiodarone
Sotalol	Class IB	Amiodarone	Sotalol
Class IA	Sotalol	Class IA	Class IA
	Class IC		
	Class IA		
	Amiodarone		

*Drugs are listed in decreasing order of choice.
†Atrial tachycardia, atrial fibrillation, and atrial flutter.
‡Complex ventricular ectopy, ventricular tachycardia, and ventricular fibrillation.

should never be used. For ventricular arrhythmias, the primary consideration in patients without underlying heart disease (i.e., patients in whom the risk for sudden death is usually very low) is to be sure not to increase the risk of death by exposing the patients to the risk of proarrhythmia. Thus, in choosing drug therapy, one should err on the side of safety; Class II and Class IB drugs should be considered despite their limited effectiveness. As soon as one moves beyond these two classes of drugs, one begins accepting a substantial risk of proarrhythmia or other significant toxicity. On the other hand, for patients with underlying heart disease who require therapy for ventricular arrhythmias, efficacy (which here includes avoiding proarrhythmia) is often the primary consideration. Thus, amiodarone is often the first drug considered despite its potential for causing long-term end-organ toxicity. In the last column of Table 10.3, for drugs listed as secondary choices after amiodarone, not only do the odds of efficacy decrease but the risk of proarrhythmia increases.

To summarize, when it comes to using antiarrhythmic drugs, there are no pretty choices. The best choice is to avoid them altogether. If this is not possible, one must proceed with the goals of treatment clearly in mind and take every precaution to avoid producing more problems than are caused by the arrhythmias being treated.

CHAPTER 11

Treatment of supraventricular tachyarrhythmias

Traditionally, clinicians have tended to divide the supraventricular tachyarrhythmias into two broad categories: paroxysmal atrial tachycardia (PAT) and atrial flutter and atrial fibrillation. The term PAT has fallen into disfavor of late (it is an artifact of the days before the mechanisms of supraventricular arrhythmias were understood), but this bimodal categorization of supraventricular arrhythmias still lends itself nicely to a discussion of therapy.

Paroxysmal atrial tachycardia

PAT is a term used to describe regular supraventricular tachyarrhythmias that occur with sudden onset and terminate equally suddenly. Thus, PAT is a catchall phrase that incorporates virtually all reentrant supraventricular arrhythmias except atrial fibrillation and atrial flutter. More than 50% of PATs are caused by atrioventricular (AV) nodal reentrant tachycardia, and approximately 40% are caused by macroreentrant tachycardia mediated by an overt or concealed bypass tract. The remaining 10% or so of PATs are caused by reentrant atrial tachycardia or sinoatrial (SA) nodal reentrant tachycardia (see Chapter 1 for a description of the mechanisms of supraventricular arrhythmias).

The acute and chronic therapies of PAT are listed in Table 11.1. Acute therapy is aimed at terminating an episode of PAT. In general, this is easy to achieve. Since the AV node or the SA node is an integral part of the reentrant circuit in 90–95% of PATs (the exception is reentrant atrial tachycardia, an arrhythmia that can usually be recognized by the presence of an unusual P-wave axis), maneuvers or drugs that produce transient SA nodal or AV nodal block are

Table 11.1 Acute and chronic treatment of PAT

Acute treatment
  Goal: Termination of the arrhythmia
    Step 1: Vagal maneuvers, such as Valsalva (may be tried by the patient before
      seeking medical attention)
    Step 2: Intravenous administration of adenosine or verapamil
    Termination by antitachycardia pacing or DC cardioversion (rarely necessary)
      Chronic treatment
  Goal: Prevention of recurrences
    Infrequent or easy-to-terminate recurrences—no specific chronic therapy may
      be necessary
    Other types of recurrences
      Treatment of choice—EP testing with RF ablation to abolish reentry
      Drug therapy—one or more of several drugs may be tried empirically (see
        Table 10.2)

EP, electrophysiologic; RF, radiofrequency.

highly effective in terminating supraventricular arrhythmias. Many patients who have recurrent PAT can therefore terminate episodes themselves by performing maneuvers that cause a sudden increase in vagal tone. Such maneuvers include Valsalva, carotid massage, ocular massage, and dunking one's face in ice water. If pharmacologic intervention is necessary, the treatment of choice is intravenous adenosine, which is virtually always effective—in fact, if adenosine fails to terminate the arrhythmia, the diagnosis of PAT needs to be seriously reconsidered. Intravenous verapamil is also highly effective. Other AV nodal blocking drugs (digoxin and beta blockers) are effective but have a much longer onset of action and, once loaded, their effect persists. Unless these drugs are being administered for chronic use, they are almost never given for acute treatment of PAT. Antitachycardia pacing techniques are also highly effective in terminating supraventricular arrhythmias, but since so many less invasive options are available, pacing is rarely used unless an atrial pacemaker is already in place.

The chronic therapy for PAT has undergone a revolution in recent decades. Prior to the 1990s, pharmacologic therapy was the only viable option for most patients. Although the choices of drug therapy for the chronic treatment of PAT are broad and include all AV nodal blocking agents (beta blockers, calcium blockers, and digoxin) and Class IA, Class IC, and Class III antiarrhythmic drugs, in earlier days many of these patients were asked to take potentially toxic drugs every day to prevent non-life-threatening arrhythmias that might otherwise occur only infrequently. Given that choice, many patients quite reasonably opted for no therapy at all and accepted the fact that they would have to make periodic pilgrimages to emergency rooms to terminate acute episodes.

Fortunately, patients no longer have to make such a choice. Once the mechanisms of the arrhythmias that cause PAT finally became understood, and with parallel advances in technology, virtually all forms of PAT became curable by the technique of transcatheter ablation. With this technique, critical components of the reentrant pathways responsible for a patient's arrhythmia can be mapped in the electrophysiology catheterization laboratory and cauterized (usually with radiofrequency energy) directly through the electrophysiology catheter. The success rate for curing AV nodal reentrant tachycardias and tachycardias mediated by bypass tracts (i.e, for the vast majority of PATs) is well in excess of 95%. SA nodal reentry and intra-atrial reentry can be cured with a somewhat lower rate of success, but these arrhythmias are rare. Today, patients with almost any form of PAT should be referred for ablation if chronic drug therapy of any type is being considered.

Atrial fibrillation and atrial flutter

Atrial fibrillation and atrial flutter are fundamentally different from most of the arrhythmias that cause PAT because they arise in the atrial myocardium itself, and therefore do not require either the AV node or the SA node for their initiation or continuation. Atrial fibrillation and atrial flutter can persist in the presence of a non-functioning SA node or complete AV block. Therefore, the measures commonly used to terminate PAT (i.e., producing transient AV nodal block through vagal maneuvers or by drug administration) do not work with atrial fibrillation and atrial flutter. Drugs that can terminate these arrhythmias and prevent recurrence must necessarily act on the atrial myocardium, namely, the Class IA, Class IC, and Class III antiarrhythmic drugs. Therefore, treatment aimed at maintaining sinus rhythm is inherently difficult and relatively risky. Often, it is more appropriate to accept a "lesser" therapeutic goal—that is, to allow the underlying arrhythmia to persist while controlling the ventricular rate.

Table 11.2 Common underlying causes of atrial fibrillation and atrial flutter

Underlying heart disease
  Valvular and congenital heart disease
  Hypertensive heart disease
  Acute ischemia or infarction
  Cardiomyopathic diseases
  Pericarditis
Systemic disorders
  Hyperthyroidism
  Acute pulmonary disease
  Acute ethanol ingestion ("holiday heart")
  Stimulant administration or ingestion (e.g., caffeine, amphetamines,
    and theophylline)

Unlike arrhythmias that cause PAT, atrial fibrillation and atrial flutter often are related to an underlying disease process. The treatment of these arrhythmias, therefore, should include a systematic search for a primary cause. Table 11.2 lists the common underlying causes of atrial fibrillation and atrial flutter.

Arrhythmias caused by systemic processes (electrolyte disturbances, hyperthyroidism, pulmonary disease, and use of alcohol or stimulant drugs) often improve or disappear once the systemic process is addressed. Arrhythmias associated with underlying heart disease, on the other hand, often persist even when therapy of heart disease is optimized.

Consequences

Atrial fibrillation and atrial flutter have three major consequences that must be taken into consideration when planning therapy: loss of the atrial kick, the rapid heart rate itself, and the risk of thromboembolism (Table 11.3).

Loss of atrial kick

The function of atrial contraction is to boost diastolic pressure within the ventricles just before ventricular systole begins. End-diastolic pressure (EDP) is of paramount importance in determining the force of ventricular contraction and, therefore, of ventricular stroke volume. EDP is so important that, in general, homeostatic mechanisms work to maintain it regardless of whether there is an atrial kick. The importance of the atrial kick in maintaining adequate EDP directly

Table 11.3 Major consequences of atrial fibrillation

Loss of atrial kick
   Major hemodynamic compromise in patients with poor LV compliance
      (i.e., patients with ventricular hypertrophy)
   Mild-to-moderate hemodynamic compromise in patients with normal LV
      compliance
   Minimal-to-mild hemodynamic compromise in patients with increased LV
      compliance (i.e., patients with dilated cardiomyopathies)
Tachycardia
   Significant symptoms (palpitations and cardiac ischemia if CAD is present)
   Tachycardiomyopathy (weakening of ventricular myocardium from chronic
      tachycardia)
Thrombus formation
   Stroke or other manifestations of thromboembolic disorder

CAD, coronary artery disease; LV, left ventricle.

depends on the relative compliance, or "stiffness," of the ventricle. The atrial kick is vitally important in patients whose ventricles are noncompliant (i.e., stiff), a condition that occurs in the setting of ventricular hypertrophy, whether the hypertrophy has been caused by aortic stenosis, hypertension, or idiopathic hypertrophic cardiomyopathy. In these patients, a very high EDP is necessary to maintain an adequate stroke volume, and the high EDP is provided, at the last instant of diastole, by the atrial kick. If the atrial kick is lost (e.g., because of the onset of atrial fibrillation), the only way to achieve an adequate EDP is to raise the *mean* diastolic pressure, that is, the pressure throughout diastole—and this is what exactly happens. Because the heart's compensatory mechanisms attempt to maintain the EDP regardless of whether or not there is an atrial kick, the mean diastolic pressure suddenly rises and pulmonary congestion ensues. Thus, patients with poor ventricular compliance develop severe symptoms almost immediately if atrial fibrillation occurs; atrial kick is vital in these patients.

On the other hand, patients with dilated cardiomyopathies have enlarged, "baggy" ventricles that are significantly more compliant than normal. In these patients, the atrial kick contributes relatively little to EDP because the relatively small volume of blood provided by atrial contraction boosts pressure only slightly in a highly compliant ventricle. These patients tend to have relatively little change in their baseline symptoms with the onset of atrial fibrillation, and they often are unable to perceive any difference, at least acutely, between sinus rhythm and atrial fibrillation.

Patients with normal ventricular compliance tend to experience intermediate symptoms with the onset of atrial fibrillation. With the loss of the atrial kick, their EDP is maintained by a rise in mean diastolic pressure, but generally the elevations are not sufficient to produce pulmonary edema. These patients can usually pinpoint the time of onset of atrial fibrillation, but in most cases, their symptoms are limited to palpitations and a mild-to-moderate sensation of breathlessness.

Tachycardia

In patients with normal AV conduction, tachycardia ensues immediately with the onset of atrial fibrillation or atrial flutter. The transient decrease in stroke volume resulting from the loss of the atrial kick is partially compensated by an increase in sympathetic tone, which directly increases the heart rate and frequently also causes a sensation of anxiety. The anxiety, in turn, further increases sympathetic tone. Thus, it is not unusual for a patient with acute atrial fibrillation or atrial flutter to present with very rapid heart rates and to experience extreme palpitations. In general, however, sympathetic tone drops within a few hours, and the heart rate slows to more reasonable levels.

If heart rates remain elevated chronically—for a period of weeks or months—a tachycardiomyopathy may develop. Tachycardiomyopathy refers to the ventricular dysfunction resulting from a persistently elevated heart rate. Although relatively uncommon, this condition is indistinguishable from other forms of dilated cardiomyopathy. Fortunately, tachycardiomyopathy is largely reversible if the rapid heart rate is brought under control. In any case, the rapid heart rates accompanying atrial fibrillation and atrial flutter have significance beyond merely producing palpitations.

Thromboembolism

Perhaps the major hemodynamic consequence of atrial fibrillation (and to a lesser extent, atrial flutter) is the risk of thromboembolism. One-third of patients with chronic atrial fibrillation eventually experience stroke, and approximately 75% of those strokes are thought to be embolic in nature. Both the incidence of atrial fibrillation itself and the yearly risk of stroke in patients with atrial fibrillation increase with age. Atrial fibrillation is seen in approximately 3% of patients who are of age 60, but in more than 10% of those 80 and older. The yearly risk of stroke in 60-year-old patients with atrial fibrillation is approximately 2%, whereas that yearly risk increases to more than 5% in patients 80 or older. Furthermore, for reasons that are poorly understood, strokes that occur in patients with atrial fibrillation are more likely to cause disability and mortality than do strokes occurring in other patients. Antiembolic therapy with warfarin, or to a lesser extent with aspirin, has been shown to significantly reduce the risk of stroke in many patients with chronic atrial fibrillation. We will discuss indications for anticoagulation below.

Treating atrial fibrillation and atrial flutter

When treating atrial fibrillation and atrial flutter, there are two basic decisions that have to be made. First, should the patient receive therapy aimed at restoring and maintaining sinus rhythm (rhythm control), or instead should the patient be allowed to remain in the tachyarrhythmia, with therapeutic efforts being directed at controlling the ventricular response (rate control)? And second, what should be done to minimize the risk of stroke or other thromboembolic events?

Rhythm control versus rate control

Until a few years ago, most cardiologists assumed that patients with atrial fibrillation would have improved outcomes if they could be converted to and maintained in normal sinus rhythm. However, two major randomized clinical trials have now shown that, at least using currently available antiarrhythmic drug therapy, patients with atrial fibrillation actually had better outcomes with rate control only.

Both the Atrial Fibrillation Follow-up Investigation of Rhythm Management (AFFIRM) trial [1] and the Rate Control versus Electrical Cardioversion (RACE) trial [2] randomized patients with atrial fibrillation to therapy with either rhythm control using antiarrhythmic drugs or rate control only. Both studies showed a nearly significant trend toward worse outcomes with rhythm control. Rhythm control with antiarrhythmic drugs yielded an increase in the primary end point of death in the AFFIRM trial and an increased incidence of a primary composite end point (including death, heart failure, thromboembolism, bleeding, requirement for a pacemaker, and severe adverse drug reactions) in the RACE trial. In neither study was the quality of life improved with rhythm control. Possibly more importantly, the incidence of thromboembolism was not reduced with rhythm control.

Experts and guidelines committees have concluded, from these and other recent trials, that for most patients with atrial fibrillation, the rate-control approach is more appropriate. The use of antiarrhythmic drugs to try to maintain sinus rhythm should generally be limited to patients who have persistent symptoms of shortness of breath, palpitations, heart failure, or angina despite adequate rate control, or for those in whom adequate rate control cannot be attained, or for patients who, after being fully informed of the risks and benefits, opt for rhythm control themselves.

It has been speculated that the negative results reported by the AF-FIRM and RACE trials regarding the strategy of rhythm control have mostly to do with the use of antiarrhythmic drugs, which are only partially effective in maintaining sinus rhythm and which themselves can cause significant toxicity. Electrophysiologists, in particular, tend to subscribe to the theory that restoring sinus rhythm by discovering and applying appropriate ablation techniques would yield different results from these two trials. While there is at least a reasonable chance that these experts are correct, at this point no study has shown that atrial fibrillation ablation procedures lead to better overall outcomes or reduce the risk of thromboembolism.

Catheter-based ablation techniques aimed at restoring and maintaining sinus rhythm in patients with atrial fibrillation are still in the developmental stages, and the efficacy for ablation for atrial fibrillation is still relatively limited, while complications are nontrivial. In contrast, transcatheter ablation techniques are quite effective at eliminating atrial flutter and are acceptably safe. For this reason, antiarrhythmic drugs are used only rarely in the chronic management of atrial flutter.

Cardioversion in atrial fibrillation and atrial flutter
There are at least two circumstances in which it is desirable to convert patients from atrial fibrillation or atrial flutter back to normal sinus rhythm. The first is when a rhythm-control strategy has been decided upon, and the second is when patients present with paroxysmal atrial fibrillation or atrial flutter.

Paroxysmal atrial fibrillation and atrial flutter have been defined as arrhythmias that have been present for less than 7 days (though most paroxysmal atrial fibrillation persists for less than 24 h). By definition, then, patients who have paroxysmal episodes of atrial fibrillation or atrial flutter are usually in sinus rhythm. Therefore, the primary goal of therapy in these patients ought to be to restore normal sinus rhythm, and to do so within 24 hours of the onset of the arrhythmia (to avoid the likelihood of formation of atrial thrombi).

In most patients presenting with paroxysmal atrial fibrillation and atrial flutter, the arrhythmias will spontaneously revert to sinus rhythm within a few hours of onset. Thus, in most instances, one merely needs to control the heart rate and wait. However, if the arrhythmia persists for 24 hours, elective cardioversion should be performed. If the patient has not presented for medical care until the arrhythmia has persisted for more than 48 hours, cardioversion should be postponed until 4 weeks of anticoagulation with warfarin has been accomplished; warfarin should also be continued for 4 weeks after cardioversion.

There are two methods for converting patients back to sinus rhythm—direct-current (DC) cardioversion or pharmacologic cardioversion. DC cardioversion has a much higher efficacy rate and is not proarrhythmic, and is the generally preferred method. If drug therapy is chosen for cardioversion, propafenone, flecainide, ibutilide, and dofetilide have been shown to be effective in restoring sinus rhythm in up to 60% of patients.

Rate control in atrial fibrillation

For patients who remain in chronic atrial fibrillation or atrial flutter, controlling the ventricular response is important. Rapid ventricular rates lead to symptoms of palpitations, easy fatigue, breathlessness, and poor exercise capacity. Persistent tachycardia can also lead to cardiomyopathy.

In most patients, rate control can be achieved by the use of beta blockers and verapamil or diltiazem. Especially in patients with heart failure, digoxin may also be helpful in slowing the ventricular response. Amiodarone is effective in slowing the ventricular response during chronic atrial fibrillation but is not used commonly for this purpose because of its impressive toxicity. (The investigational drug dronedarone, a "cousin" of amiodarone discussed in Chapter 8, also appears effective for this purpose and so far, appears to have much less end-organ toxicity.)

Achieving adequate rate control means controlling the heart rate both at rest and during exercise. The average resting heart rate should be less than 80 beats/min, and during moderate ambulation, it should be less than 110 beats/min. The overall average heart rate during 24-hour Holter monitoring should be less than 100 beats/min.

Titration of rate-control measures can be made by observing the resting and exercise heart rates. Calcium blockers tend to slow the heart rate at rest, while beta blockers tend to be more effective in slowing the heart rate during exercise. Often, a combination of drugs is required, established by means of a trial-and-error approach.

Adequate rate control can be achieved in the large majority of patients with pharmacologic therapy. However, occasional patients cannot tolerate adequate doses of beta blockers, calcium blockers, or digoxin to achieve control. In these patients, strong consideration ought to be given to transcatheter ablation of the AV junction to achieve complete heart block and the insertion of a permanent pacemaker. This technique, while irreversible and seemingly somewhat drastic, is actually relatively simple to perform and is very effective and reasonably safe.

Rhythm control in atrial fibrillation

Whenever maintaining sinus rhythm is the goal of therapy, selecting an appropriate antiarrhythmic drug requires consideration of the available drugs themselves (i.e., their likely efficacy and toxicity), as well as the clinical status of the patient being treated. It should be kept in mind that, according to the best available data, a rhythm-control strategy does not improve patients' outcomes and further, does not preclude the need for long-term anticoagulation. Thus, in most cases, the aim of a rhythm-control strategy is merely to reduce the incidence and perhaps the severity of symptomatic episodes of atrial fibrillation.

In general, six antiarrhythmic agents are primarily used today in a rhythm-control strategy: disopyramide (Class IA), flecainide and propafenone (Class IC), and sotalol, dofetilide, and amiodarone (Class III). Table 11.4 lists the drugs of choice according to the 2006 guidelines from the American College of Cardiology/American Heart Association/European Society of Cardiology (ACC/AHA/ESC).

The general consensus of cardiologists, backed up by increasing clinical evidence, is that amiodarone is the most effective antiarrhythmic drug available for maintaining sinus rhythm after cardioversion from atrial fibrillation. Furthermore, it has a relatively low incidence of proarrhythmia, even in patients with underlying heart disease. However, amiodarone carries the significant baggage

Table 11.4 Antiarrhythmic drugs for rhythm control in atrial fibrillation

Patients with no structural heart disease (or with hypertension without LVH)
1st choice—propafenone, flecainide, and sotalol
2nd choice—amiodarone, dofetilide, and ablation
Patients with heart failure or significant LV dysfunction
1st choice—amiodarone and dofetilide
2nd choice—ablation
Patients with coronary artery disease
1st choice—sotalol and dofetilide
2nd choice—amiodarone or ablation
Patients with hypertension with LVH
1st choice—amiodarone
2nd choice—ablation
Special cases
Vagally mediated atrial fibrillation—disopyramide
Adrenergically mediated atrial fibrillation—beta blockers

LV, left ventricular; LVH, left ventricular hypertrophy.

of having a truly impressive array of potential end-organ toxicities—not to mention the fact that its use for atrial fibrillation is not approved by the FDA—and it ought to be reserved, in general, for patients whose hemodynamic compromise while in atrial fibrillation is severe and in whom other antiarrhythmic drugs are not effective or safe. The 2006 guidelines from the ACC/AHA/ESC recommended that amiodarone be used as first-line therapy only in patients with heart failure or significant left ventricular systolic dysfunction, or in patients with hypertension and left ventricular hypertrophy. (Left ventricular hypertrophy, like systolic dysfunction, is often associated with underlying electrophysiologic abnormalities that increase the risk of proarrhythmia with other antiarrhythmic drugs.)

Flecainide and propafenone are reasonably effective in maintaining sinus rhythm, but because of their proarrhythmic potential they should be used only in patients with no structural heart disease, and who do not have coronary artery disease (or for that matter, a high risk of developing coronary artery disease).

Sotalol and dofetilide are also moderately effective. These drugs do not exacerbate reentrant arrhythmias (like the Class IC drugs do), and as long as appropriate cautions are taken to reduce the incidence of torsades de pointes, these are reasonably safe in patients with underlying heart disease.

Disopyramide, because of its vagolytic effects, may be effective in treating the relatively uncommon varieties of atrial fibrillation that are triggered by strong vagal stimulation (such as swallowing cold liquids).

Finally, beta blockers may be effective in preventing the recurrence of certain kinds of atrial fibrillation that seem to be induced by increased sympathetic tone.

Anticoagulation in atrial fibrillation and atrial flutter

Most often, preventing stroke should be the doctor's chief goal in treating patients with atrial fibrillation or atrial flutter. The only method that has been shown to reliably reduce the risk of stroke is anticoagulation with warfarin and, to a lesser extent, with aspirin. Thus, when seeing a patient who has atrial fibrillation or atrial flutter, the decision as to whether to anticoagulate should always be actively considered.

In 2006, the ACC/AHA/ESC published joint guidelines on the use of chronic antithrombotic therapy in patients with atrial fibrillation or atrial flutter [3]. These guidelines are fairly complex and can be difficult to sort through, but in general they can be summarized as follows:

Patients with atrial fibrillation or atrial flutter can be categorized into one of two groups: patients at low risk and patients at high risk for thromboembolism. Those in the low-risk categories should be treated with aspirin (81–325 mg/day) unless contraindicated. Those in the high-risk categories should be treated with oral anticoagulation in order to produce an INR of 2.0–3.0, unless contraindicated.

Determining whether patients fit into a low- or high-risk category depends on two general factors: age and the presence of risk factors for thromboembolism. The risk factors include heart failure, left ventricular ejection fraction <0.35, history of hypertension, valvular heart disease, diabetes, and prior history of thromboembolism.

Patients in the low-risk category include:

Age <75 and no risk factors

Patients in the high-risk category include:

Age 75 or greater,

Age <75, but presence of risk factors

While patients with paroxysmal atrial fibrillation have long been thought to have a lower incidence of embolization than those with chronic atrial fibrillation, at least two large clinical trials have now shown similar risks among these patients—and similar benefits from anticoagulation. Thus, patients with paroxysmal atrial fibrillation should be treated according to these same guidelines.

Additionally, both the AFFIRM and RACE trials have suggested that patients treated with the goal of restoring and maintaining sinus rhythm (as opposed to rate control) do not have a substantially reduced risk of thromboembolism. Accordingly, these patients should also be treated according to these guidelines.

Finally, it is by no means clear that patients with atrial fibrillation who are treated by ablation techniques in order to restore and maintain sinus rhythm will have a reduced risk of stroke. For now, chronic anticoagulation should also be strongly considered in these patients.

References

1 Wyse DG, Waldo AL, DiMarco JP, et al. A comparison of rate control and rhythm control in patients with atrial fibrillation. N Engl J Med 2002;347(23):1825.
2 Van Gelder IC, Hagens VE, Bosker HA, et al. A comparison of rate control and rhythm control in patients with recurrent persistent atrial fibrillation. N Engl J Med 2002;347(23):1834.
3 Furster V, Ryden LE, Cannom DS, et al. ACC/AHA/ESC guidelines for the management of patients with atrial fibrillation. A report of the American College of Cardiology/American Heart Association Task Force on Practice Guidelines and the European Society of Cardiology Committee for Practice Guidelines (Writing committee to revise the 2001guidelines for the management of patients with atrial fibrillation). J Am Coll Cardiol 2006;48:e149.

CHAPTER 12
Treatment of ventricular arrhythmias

Ventricular arrhythmias are responsible for hundreds of thousands of sudden deaths each year in the United States alone. Therapeutically, patients at risk for sudden death usually fall into one of the two broad categories. First, there are patients who have already experienced an episode of sustained ventricular tachycardia (VT) or ventricular fibrillation (VF). These individuals, having already demonstrated a propensity for lethal arrhythmias, are at substantial risk for subsequent sudden death. The second and much larger category consists of individuals who are at high risk but have not yet had sustained ventricular arrhythmias. These patients generally have significant underlying cardiac disease, whether or not it is accompanied by complex ventricular ectopy (consisting of frequent premature ventricular complexes (PVCs), nonsustained VT, or both). The risk of sudden death for these patients, although demonstrably increased over normal levels, is generally not as high as for patients in the first category.

Treatment of nonsustained ventricular arrhythmias

The significance of ventricular ectopy
Ventricular ectopy is generally classified as being either *simple* or *complex*. Simple ventricular ectopy is said to be present in patients who have PVCs, but fewer than 10 PVCs per hour during 24-hour Holter monitoring and no nonsustained VT. Complex ventricular ectopy is generally defined as >10 PVCs per hour during 24-hour monitoring or the presence of nonsustained VT. Simple ventricular ectopy carries no prognostic significance. However, in the presence of underlying cardiac disease, complex ventricular ectopy does have prognostic implications. Indeed, complex ectopy is relatively uncommon in

Table 12.1 Relationship of ventricular ectopy to estimated risk of sudden death

Number of risk factors	One-year risk (%)
One	
Previous MI	5
LVEF < 0.40	
Two	
Previous MI + CVE	10
LVEF <0.40 + CVE	
Previous MI + LVEF <0.40	
Three	
Previous MI + LVEF <0.40 + CVE	15

CVE, complex ventricular ectopy; LVEF, left ventricular ejection fraction; MI, myocardial infarction.

patients with normal hearts. The presence of unexpected complex ventricular ectopy should thus prompt an evaluation for undiagnosed cardiac disease.

It is possible to estimate a patient's risk of sudden death by considering the presence of three simple clinical factors: previous myocardial infarction, depressed left ventricular ejection fraction (i.e., an ejection fraction of less than 0.40), and complex ventricular ectopy. The resultant risks are shown in Table 12.1. If previous myocardial infarction or depressed ventricular function are present (as noted, the presence of complex ectopy alone carries no prognostic significance), the 1-year risk of sudden death is approximately 5%. If any two risk factors are present, the 1-year risk of sudden death is approximately 10%. If all three risk factors are present, the 1-year risk is approximately 15%. Thus, patients who have survived myocardial infarction or who have depressed ventricular function from any cause have increased risk of sudden death. The risk increases with the presence of complex ventricular ectopy.

Treating ventricular ectopy

The association between complex ectopy and the risk of sudden death has been recognized for decades, and for many years, it was assumed that antiarrhythmic drug therapy aimed at eliminating complex ectopy would improve that risk. This assumption was proven wrong in the late 1980s courtesy of the Cardiac Arrhythmia

Suppression Trial (CAST), discussed in Chapter 9. To review, CAST randomized patients who had survived myocardial infarctions and who had complex ectopy (and who, therefore had an increased risk of sudden death) either to have their ectopy suppressed with Class IC drugs or to receive placebo. Much to the surprise of many observers, and in distinct contrast to the predictions of most experts, patients whose ectopy had been successfully suppressed by the Class IC agents generally had a significant *increase* in mortality as compared to patients on placebo. Not only did getting rid of the ectopy fail to improve outcomes, but also the use of antiarrhythmic drugs itself (presumably due to proarrhythmia) increased mortality. The findings of CAST were reinforced by subsequent meta-analyses, showing that patients treated with Class I antiarrhythmic drugs commonly have reduced survival as compared to patients on placebo.

In conceptualizing the treatment of complex ventricular ectopy, the bear droppings theory is instructive—if you are walking in the woods and see bear droppings, your chances of being eaten by a bear are higher than if there were no bear droppings. However, if you take out your gun and shoot the bear droppings, you are not reducing your risk. In fact, you might even induce the bear to come by to investigate the disturbance. Complex ectopy is best viewed as an indication of increased risk (like bear droppings), and not as an indication for therapy.

The prophylactic empiric use of amiodarone has also been advanced as a way of treating patients with underlying heart disease who have complex ventricular ectopy, and several randomized trials have now examined this question. The results of the trials are summarized in Table 12.2. Unfortunately, these results do not provide definitive evidence that prophylactic use of amiodarone is helpful. In the Basel Antiarrhythmic Study of Infarct Survival (BASIS) [1], patients treated with amiodarone had improved overall mortality compared with that of control patients. In the Canadian Amiodarone Myocardial Infarction Arrhythmia Trial (CAMIAT) [2] and the European Myocardial Infarct Amiodarone Trial (EMIAT) [3], amiodarone yielded a reduction in arrhythmic death but not in overall mortality. In the Veterans Administration Congestive Heart Failure Antiarrhythmic Trial (CHF-STAT) [4], no improvement in mortality with amiodarone was seen compared with that of controls. Overall, these findings suggest that amiodarone-related toxicity may largely negate any reduction in sudden death. However, in distinct contrast to the Class I drugs, amiodarone is *not* associated with an

Table 12.2 Clinical trials examining the prophylactic use of empiric amiodarone

Trial	Patient population	Randomization	Reduction in arrhythmic or cardiac mortality*	Reduction in total mortality*
BASIS	MI, CVE	amio 200 mg/day vs. other drugs or placebo	—	Yes
CHF-STAT	low EF, CVE	amio 200 mg/day vs. placebo	—	No
CAMIAT	MI, CVE	amio 300 mg/day vs. placebo	Yes	No
EMIAT	MI, low EF	amio 200 mg/day vs. placebo	Yes	No

*Reduction in indicated mortality with amiodarone versus controls.
BASIS, Basel Antiarrhythmic Study of Infarct Survival; CHF-STAT, Veterans Administration Congestive Heart Failure Antiarrhythmic Trial; CAMIAT, Canadian Amiodarone Myocardial Infarction Arrhythmia Trial; EMIAT, European Myocardial Infarct Amiodarone Trial; amio, amiodarone; CVE, complex ventricular ectopy; EF, left ventricular ejection fraction; MI, myocardial infarction.

increase in mortality when used in patients with complex ectopy and underlying heart disease.

The bottom line is that treating ventricular ectopy with antiarrhythmic drugs has not been associated with an improved clinical outcome, despite the fact that numerous clinical trials have been conducted to examine this question. Therefore, it is not appropriate to treat these patients with antiarrhythmic drugs for the purpose of improving their survival.

However, on occasion, it may be appropriate to treat ventricular ectopy if the ectopic beats themselves are producing significant symptoms. Here, obviously, the goal is to improve symptoms (and not necessarily to abolish the ectopy completely). In general, when trying to suppress ventricular ectopy for the purpose of relieving symptoms, the appropriate choice of an antiarrhythmic drug depends on the patient's clinical condition.

In patients with no underlying heart disease, beta blockers should be the first drugs attempted, since they are well tolerated and have relatively few side effects. Unfortunately, they are also generally ineffective in suppressing ventricular ectopy. The use of flecainide might be a reasonable option, since the drug is reasonably well tolerated, is quite effective at suppressing ectopy, and should have little proarrhythmic potential in patients with structurally normal hearts and a low risk of developing ischemic heart disease. However, because of the results of CAST, some experts are reluctant to recommend flecainide (or any Class IC drug) for the treatment of ventricular ectopy in any patients, no matter how healthy he or she appears to be. Sotalol and dofetilide may be reasonable choices if beta blockers are ineffective (despite the fact that their efficacy in suppressing ventricular ectopy is not well documented), but precautions must be taken with these Class III agents to minimize the risk of torsades de pointes. Finally, amiodarone can be considered—but its ability to suppress symptomatic ectopy needs to be carefully weighed against its propensity to cause end-organ toxicities that might well dwarf the significance of palpitations.

In patients with underlying heart disease who need to be treated to reduce symptomatic ventricular ectopy, beta blockers are a clear first choice, since these drugs need to be used anyway in patients with prior myocardial infarctions or heart failure (because of the significant improvement in survival they impart to these patients). If the ventricular ectopy remains a problem, amiodarone can be considered, as well as sotalol or dofetilide.

Treatment of sustained ventricular arrhythmias

Patients who have survived an episode of sustained VT or VF have an extraordinarily high risk of experiencing a recurrent arrhythmia. In general, 30–50% will have another episode of sustained ventricular tachyarrhythmia within 2 years. Therefore, once such an arrhythmia has occurred, aggressive measures must be taken to reduce the subsequent risk of sudden death.

Treatment of sustained monomorphic VT

Most patients presenting with sustained monomorphic VT (i.e., regular VT with a stable QRS complex, occurring at a rate of more than 100 beats/min, and persisting for at least 30 s) are survivors of myocardial infarction. Sustained monomorphic VT in any patient is usually a strong indicator that a fixed reentrant circuit exists within the ventricular myocardium, and thus, once seen, monomorphic VT is likely to recur.

Most episodes of sustained monomorphic VT occur after the acute phase of a myocardial infarction, that is, after the first 48 hours, and usually within the first year, but sometimes as late as several years after acute myocardial damage occurs. The prognosis of patients with monomorphic VT is relatively poor, largely because this arrhythmia tends to be associated with poor left ventricular function, heart failure, and multivessel coronary artery disease. While most episodes of VF are preceded by at least short episodes of VT, it is not clear that patients presenting with stable, sustained monomorphic VT—at least those who survive and are referred to electrophysiologists—have an extraordinarily high risk of subsequent VF. The incidence of sudden death in patients presenting with well-tolerated monomorphic VT is substantially lower than that for patients who have survived cardiac arrest, though their overall rate of subsequent mortality (probably due to the extent of underlying heart disease) remains elevated.

Acute treatment

Patients presenting with sustained monomorphic VT can be treated acutely with direct-current (DC) cardioversion or with intravenous antiarrhythmic drugs. Intravenous procainamide is often useful (i.e., effective in up to 50% of patients) in terminating hemodynamically stable VT. Intravenous amiodarone can also be used, and is especially useful for controlling sustained VT that is recurring frequently. Intravenous lidocaine, for decades the drug of choice, is now felt to be only marginally effective in terminating monomorphic VT, unless the arrhythmia is being caused by active myocardial ischemia.

Chronic treatment

Monomorphic VT in the setting of underlying heart disease is almost always a reentrant arrhythmia. Unfortunately, it is difficult to predict the effect of a particular antiarrhythmic drug on a particular reentrant circuit. The same drug may have a beneficial effect on one circuit but a proarrhythmic effect on another. Ideally, some means should be used to measure the effect of a drug before a patient is committed to long-term therapy. Two general methods of guiding drug therapy have been used in patients with ventricular tachyarrhythmias: Holter monitoring and electrophysiologic (EP) testing.

Holter monitoring was the only methodology available for guiding drug therapy until the late 1970s, and it was widely used until almost 1990. The use of this method relied on the suppression of ambient ventricular ectopy, but as we have seen, this technique was rendered a death blow by the CAST study.

The idea behind EP testing to guide drug therapy is essentially sound, at least in theory. If a reentrant circuit is present that is capable of generating an arrhythmia, all you need to do to start the arrhythmia is to introduce an appropriately timed electrical impulse into the circuit (see Figure 1.7). This procedure can be accomplished in the EP laboratory by the technique known as programmed stimulation, in which a temporary ventricular pacemaker is used to deliver precisely timed, paced impulses into a presumed reentrant circuit. If such a circuit exists and if it has the appropriate EP characteristics (as discussed in Chapter 1), VT can be induced.

EP testing, therefore, can help to determine whether a reentrant circuit capable of generating a ventricular tachyarrhythmia is present. Among patients presenting with sustained monomorphic VT, the presumed clinical arrhythmia can be induced in approximately 90%. Sustained VT can also be induced in 30–60% of patients whose presenting arrhythmia is VF. In addition to assessing the presence or absence of a reentrant circuit, EP testing can be used in the attempt to assess the effect that an antiarrhythmic drug might have on the reentrant circuit. The assessment is done by administering one of the antiarrhythmic drugs and then attempting to reinduce the arrhythmia. If a previously inducible arrhythmia is rendered noninducible by a drug, it is assumed that the drug has favorably changed the characteristics of the reentrant circuit. Chronic therapy with the drug then seems reasonable.

This kind of EP testing was widely used by electrophysiologists from the early 1980s until the mid-1990s in guiding the therapy of patients presenting with sustained monomorphic VT. But clinical reports by the mid-1990s began to call into question the ability of such "EP-guided" therapy to actually improve the outcomes of patients with this arrhythmia VT. This growing skepticism was finally confirmed by the Electrophysiologic Testing Versus Electrocardiographic Monitoring (ESVEM) trial [5]. In ESVEM, patients presenting with sustained VT, who also had both a high degree of ambient ventricular ectopy and inducible VT, were randomized to drug therapy guided by either EP testing or Holter monitoring. Both groups had very similar, and very poor, outcomes. The rate of recurrent arrhythmias for both treatment groups was nearly 40% at 1 year and 66% at 4 years. This trial convinced most electrophysiologists that EP-guided drug testing is no more effective in improving clinical outcomes than is Holter-guided drug testing. Neither method works adequately, and we now know that neither should be relied upon to direct therapy in patients presenting with VT.

Empiric drug therapy

Using antiarrhythmic drugs empirically simply means administering them without an attempt to measure their efficacy beforehand. Empiric drug therapy as the primary treatment for ventricular tachyarrhythmias was common before 1980, but was deemed unacceptable with the advent of EP testing. By the time EP testing also fell out of favor in the late 1990s, the phenomenon of proarrhythmia with Class I antiarrhythmic drugs was widely recognized, rendering the idea of simply going back to empiric therapy (at least with most antiarrhythmic drugs), generally unacceptable as the primary approach to treating patients with sustained VT.

However, empiric therapy with antiarrhythmic drugs can be useful as a supplement to patients who have received implantable cardioverter defibrillators (ICDs), or in patients who refuse to receive or are not good candidates for one of these devices. Because they have a relatively low propensity to exacerbate reentrant VT, the Class III antiarrhythmic drugs today are the ones most commonly used for empiric therapy.

There is evidence from clinical trials that amiodarone, in particular, can be effective—certainly more effective than Class I drugs—in treating patients presenting with sustained VT. The Cardiac Arrest in Seattle—Conventional Versus Amiodarone Drug Evaluation (CASCADE) trial [6], in which survivors of cardiac arrest were randomized to receive either empiric treatment with amiodarone or treatment with conventional drugs guided by EP testing, Holter monitoring, or both, showed that amiodarone was significantly better than conventional drugs in reducing the incidence of cardiac mortality and recurrent arrhythmic events. Implantable defibrillators were also used in many patients in the study, so the effect of amiodarone in reducing mortality could not be well evaluated in this trial.

Other Class III agents may also reduce the risk of recurrent arrhythmias in patients presenting with sustained VT. Sotalol, in particular, seems to provide some benefit in these patients, and there is preliminary evidence that dofetilide, as well as the investigational drug azimilide, may also be helpful. Again, however, whenever possible, empiric antiarrhythmic drug therapy should be reserved for patients who have ICDs. Empiric drug therapy simply cannot be relied upon as the primary treatment of choice for patients presenting with sustained ventricular tachyarrhythmias.

Implantable cardioverter defibrillators

An ICD is a pacemakerlike device that automatically detects the onset of ventricular tachyarrhythmias and then takes action to terminate them, either by administering a DC shock to the heart (for VF or very rapid VT) or by delivering bursts of antitachycardia pacing (for slower sustained VTs). The ICD has been in clinical use since the early 1980s, and vast, worldwide experience with the device has been gathered. ICDs can now be implanted with a surgical mortality of much less than 1%, and they have proven to be extremely effective in preventing sudden death from ventricular tachyarrhythmias. Survivors of cardiac arrest, whose risk of recurrent life-threatening arrhythmias is otherwise as high as 40% after 2 years, have had the risk of sudden death reduced by the ICD to less than 2% at 1 year and less than 6% at 5 years. No other therapy is as effective in eliminating the risk of sudden death in this population.

Whether ICDs produce a significant decrease in mortality in patients presenting with relatively well-tolerated sustained monomorphic VT, however, is a somewhat more difficult question. While many, if not most, episodes of VF are preceded by at least a few beats of VT, it is unclear how often patients who have recurrent, prolonged episodes of hemodynamically stable monomorphic VT go on to develop VF. Nonetheless, there are at least two reasons to strongly consider implanting ICDs in these patients.

First, ICDs can often terminate monomorphic VT by means of their (painless) antitachycardia pacing algorithms, thus restoring normal sinus rhythm without the need for painful shocks. And second, the large majority of patients presenting with monomorphic VT will already have an indication for an ICD. Patients with reduced ejection fractions and either prior myocardial infarctions or a history of heart failure (i.e., the majority of patients with monomorphic VT) have now been shown to have significantly improved survival with ICDs, regardless of whether or not they have had prior ventricular arrhythmias. Most patients with monomorphic VT, therefore, will already fit widely accepted criteria for implantation of an ICD.

Treatment of hemodynamically unstable VT or VF

The chief clinical goal in treating patients who have survived ventricular tachyarrhythmias that produced hemodynamic instability—that is, patients who have survived cardiac arrest—is to reduce their high residual risk of sudden death. Several randomized clinical trials have now shown that in these patients the ICD produces a significant reduction in mortality, of up to 25%, as compared to antiarrhythmic drugs, including amiodarone. Guidelines from the American College of Cardiology/American Heart Association/Heart Rhythm Society now recommend the ICD for survivors of cardiac arrest, unless the cardiac arrest was due to transient or reversible causes.

If an ICD cannot be used for some reason, empiric therapy with amiodarone appears to offer at least some protection from recurrent cardiac arrest and should be considered. In addition, beta blockers have been shown to reduce the risk of sudden death in both survivors of myocardial infarction and patients with heart failure, and they should be given to these patients whether they have had sustained ventricular arrhythmias or not.

As already noted, Class III antiarrhythmic drugs are frequently useful as adjunctive therapy in patients who have ICDs as a means of reducing the need for shocks. However, since these drugs (especially amiodarone) have been reported to occasionally increase the threshold for defibrillation, potentially rendering the ICD less effective, and because they (again, especially amiodarone) can cause significant toxicity, their use as adjunctive therapy in patients with ICDs should not be taken lightly.

Treatment of less common forms of ventricular tachyarrhythmias

In Chapter 1, we mentioned several less common forms of ventricular tachyarrhythmias, none of which are caused by the typical intramyocardial reentrant circuits associated with coronary artery disease or cardiomyopathy. Two of these are known to be due to channelopathies—the arrhythmias caused by triggered activity, and those related to the Brugada syndrome—and were covered in some detail in the discussion on channelopathies in that chapter. The remaining uncommon forms of VT will now be discussed in more detail.

VT associated with right ventricular dysplasia

"Arrhythmogenic" right ventricular dysplasia (AVRD) is a condition of unknown etiology, most commonly seen in younger individuals, characterized by the replacement of the right ventricular myocardium with fibrofatty tissue, and the propensity to develop ventricular tachyarrhythmias. Sustained monomorphic VT originating in the right ventricle (and thus having a left bundle branch block pattern to the QRS complexes) is the most common presenting arrhythmia, but sudden death (especially during exercise) can be the first presenting symptom. The arrhythmias seen with AVRD are related to reentrant circuits that arise as a result of the fibrofatty deposits.

Treatment of these VTs generally consists of either drug therapy with sotalol (which has been reported to suppress arrhythmias associated with AVRD in over 60% of patients) or amiodarone, or with an ICD. ICD usage is often supplemented with antiarrhythmic drug therapy.

Drug therapy alone should generally be reserved for patients who have had well-tolerated, sustained monomorphic VT, since these patients are thought to have a relatively low risk of sudden death. ICDs should be chosen as primary therapy for higher-risk patients, a category that includes younger patients, those presenting with syncope, presyncope, or cardiac arrest, or those with a family history of cardiac arrest or syncope related to this condition.

Bundle branch reentry

Bundle branch reentry is seen occasionally in patients with dilated cardiomyopathy and intraventricular conduction delays. While such patients, due to the nature of their underlying heart disease, have a high propensity for "typical" reentrant ventricular arrhythmias, they can also develop bundle branch reentry. In bundle branch reentry, the reentrant circuit is formed by the right and left bundle branches, the bundle of His, and the intervening ventricular myocardium. An arrhythmia can be triggered when a premature ventricular impulse enters both bundle branches in the retrograde direction, is blocked in the right bundle branch but conducts up the left bundle branch (which has a shorter refractory period) and then turns around at the bundle of His and reenters the right bundle branch in the antegrade direction. The resulting VT will therefore have a left bundle branch block configuration. It is often a very rapid VT that causes hemodynamic instability.

Radiofrequency ablation of the right bundle branch completely eliminates this arrhythmia, and is considered the treatment of choice by many electrophysiologists. However, these patients almost always have a markedly reduced left ventricular ejection fraction and a history of heart failure, and therefore are indicated for ICDs even if their bundle branch reentry is "cured." Ablation of the bundle branch reentry circuit, then, ought to be thought of, in most cases, as an adjunctive therapy, aimed at reducing the need for ICD shocks. Antiarrhythmic drugs have little or no role in the management of bundle branch reentry.

Repetitive monomorphic VT

Repetitive monomorphic VT (RMVT), also known as right ventricular outflow tract tachycardia, presents as bursts of nonsustained, monomorphic VT with a left bundle branch block pattern and an inferior axis. These arrhythmias originate, for the most part, in the outflow tract of the right ventricle. They are seen almost exclusively in young-to-middle-age patients, and they are exacerbated by increased adrenergic tone. Patients with RMVT most often present with complaints of palpitations or light-headedness associated with exercise or emotional stress. In addition, women with RMVT will often complain of the same symptoms during certain times of the menstrual cycle. While sudden death is not unheard of in patients with RMVT, its incidence is thought to be quite low.

There is now evidence that at least some cases of RMVT may be related to a form of triggered activity that produces delayed afterdepolarizations (see Chapter 1). In any case, RMVT tends to respond to antiarrhythmic drugs that are generally ineffective in treating more typical forms of VT, including adenosine, verapamil, and beta blockers. Class I and Class III antiarrhythmic drugs are also effective reasonably often. However, since these arrhythmias are often localizable, they are quite amenable to radiofrequency ablation, which is reported to be completely effective in over 80% of cases.

There is a condition often referred to as "paroxysmal sustained VT," which is virtually identical to RMVT (including its response to verapamil and adenosine) except that the episodes of VT persist for much longer than the dozen or so beats usually seen with RMVT. Some experts consider this a distinct syndrome, while others consider it simply an exaggerated form of RMVT.

Idiopathic left ventricular tachycardia

Idiopathic left ventricular tachycardia (ILVT) is another form of VT associated with young patients who have no identifiable underlying heart disease. These patients present with sustained VT originating from inferior-apical or mid-septal region of the left ventricle (yielding a right bundle branch block and left superior axis QRS complex). The arrhythmia is not associated with exercise, and symptoms are usually limited to palpitations and light-headedness. Sudden death in patients with ILVT is thought to be rare. Studies in electrophysiology laboratory suggest that ILVT is an unusual form of reentry, associated with abnormal Purkinje tissue that is sensitive to verapamil.

Indeed, the sensitivity of this arrhythmia to verapamil is perhaps its most distinctive feature, and chronic verapamil therapy is often very effective in suppressing ILVT. The arrhythmia is also typically quite amenable to radiofrequency ablation.

References

1 Burkart F, Pfisterer M, and Kiowski W. Effect of antiarrhythmic therapy on mortality in survivors of MI with asymptomatic complex ventricular arrhythmias. Basel Antiarrhythmic Study of Infarct Survival (BASIS). J Am Coll Cardiol 1990;16:1711.

2 Cairns JA, Connolly SJ, Roberts R, et al. Randomised trial of outcome after myocardial infarction in patients with frequent or repetitive premature depolarisations: CAMIAT. Lancet 1997;349:675.

3 Julian DG, Camm AJ, Frangin G, et al. Randomised trial of effect of amiodarone on mortality in patients with left-ventricular dysfunction after recent myocardial infarction: EMIAT. Lancet 1997;349:667.

4 Singh SN, Fletcher RD, Fisher SG, et al. Amiodarone in patients with congestive heart failure and asymptomatic ventricular arrhythmia. Survival Trial of Antiarrhythmic Therapy in Congestive Heart Failure. N Engl J Med 1995;333:77.

5 Mason JW. A comparison of electrophysiologic testing with Holter monitoring to predict antiarrhythmic drug efficacy for ventricular tachyarrhythmias. Electrophysiologic Study versus Electrocardiographic Monitoring Investigators. N Engl J Med 1993;329:445.

6 The CASCADE Investigators. Randomized antiarrhythmic drug therapy in survivors of cardiac arrest (the CASCADE study). Am J Cardiol 1993;72: 280.

CHAPTER 13

Treatment of arrhythmias in pregnancy

Pregnancy creates several types of physiologic stress, and as a result, women who are prone to develop cardiac arrhythmias are more likely to experience them when they are pregnant. These physiologic stresses include the hemodynamic stress produced by a "chronic" high-output state, various hormonal shifts, and changes in autonomic tone. Further, women with congenital heart disease, even if successfully repaired, are especially likely to develop arrhythmias if they become pregnant.

Women who have the electrophysiologic substrate for reentrant supraventricular arrhythmias—especially AV nodal reentrant tachycardia and bypass-tract-mediated tachycardia, that is, arrhythmias in which the AV node is part of the reentrant circuit—seem particularly likely to experience arrhythmias during pregnancy. This is probably due to the increased adrenergic tone that occurs in pregnant women, most often producing an increase in the resting sinus rate and a decrease in the PR interval.

Ventricular arrhythmias are relatively rare during pregnancy unless underlying heart disease is present. Indeed, women who develop ventricular arrhythmias while pregnant should be evaluated for heart disease (including pregnancy-related cardiomyopathy), as well as accelerated hypertension and thyrotoxicosis.

Using antiarrhythmic drugs in pregnancy

There is a risk to both mother and fetus in using antiarrhythmic drugs during pregnancy, and these drugs should be avoided altogether unless the arrhythmias are intolerable. Furthermore, it should be recognized that conducting systematic, prospective clinical studies on the use of antiarrhythmic drugs in pregnant women has simply not been feasible and that, therefore, the quality of information we have on the safety and efficacy of these drugs during pregnancy is quite poor and incomplete. The little that is known about the safe use of antiarrhythmic drugs during pregnancy will be summarized below.

Class IA antiarrhythmic drugs

Quinidine has been used for several decades during pregnancy, and based on this experience, it is considered to be relatively safe. In addition to the usual side effects seen with quinidine, however, fetal thrombocytopenia and premature labor have been reported.

Procainamide has not been reported to produce any problems uniquely associated with pregnancy, but many of the side effects of this drug—especially those related to immune reactions—should preclude its use.

There is little information on the use of disopyramide during pregnancy, except that it has been used to induce labor (by increasing contractions). This drug, also, should be avoided if possible.

Quinidine and disopyramide are excreted into breast milk. The American Academy of Pediatrics, however, considers these drugs to be compatible with breast-feeding.

Class IB antiarrhythmic drugs

Intravenous lidocaine appears to be safe during pregnancy, but blood levels should be monitored to avoid producing central nervous system side effects (which can affect both the mother and the fetus).

Mexiletine has not been used extensively in pregnant patients. However, hypoglycemia in the newborn has been reported after mothers have taken this drug. It is excreted into breast milk, but adverse effects to babies being breast-fed have not been reported.

Phenytoin, because of its extensive usage in the treatment of seizures, has been used for decades in pregnant women. Babies whose mothers have taken phenytoin during pregnancy have roughly twice the risk of developing congenital abnormalities as that of babies not exposed to this drug. Pregnant women on phenytoin should take folic acid each day to help prevent neural tube defects. Transient blood-clotting defects have been reported in newborns whose mothers were taking this drug, but vitamin K given to mothers during the last month of pregnancy prevents this problem. Phenytoin is excreted into breast milk in low concentrations, but it is considered safe to breast-feed full-term babies while taking this drug.

Class IC antiarrhythmic drugs

Flecainide has been used in pregnancy without adverse effects. The drug crosses the placenta and has been useful for controlling fetal supraventricular tachycardias. It is excreted into breast milk but has not been reported to cause problems in nursing infants.

Propafenone should be avoided during pregnancy because particularly little information exists about its safety. Propafenone also is excreted into breast milk but has not been recognized to cause problems to nursing babies.

Moricizine, like propafenone, has not been studied in pregnant women and should be avoided. It is excreted into breast milk, but problems to nursing babies have not been seen.

Class II antiarrhythmic drugs

Beta blockers have been used during pregnancy for decades, mainly to treat nonarrhythmic disorders such as hypertension. However, reports suggest that beta blockers may be associated with low birth weights, neonatal bradycardia and hypoglycemia. The most common antiarrhythmic application of beta blockers, in general, is to control the heart rate during atrial fibrillation. When controlling the ventricular response in atrial fibrillation during pregnancy, attempts should be made first with digoxin and verapamil, turning to beta blockers only if these are ineffective. Most beta blockers are excreted into breast milk, but it is generally considered safe to nurse full-term infants while taking beta blockers.

Class III antiarrhythmic drugs

Amiodarone is effective in treating most forms of tachyarrhythmias in both the mother and the fetus. However, its impressive end-organ toxicity and its prolonged half-life mandate that it be used only as a last resort during pregnancy. In addition to the array of "typical" amiodarone-related toxicities, risks specifically associated with pregnancy include premature labor, low birth weight, and neonatal hypothyroidism and hyperthyroidism. Amiodarone appears in breast milk, and mothers taking this drug should not breast-feed.

Sotalol has not been used widely or studied adequately during pregnancy and should be avoided. It is excreted into breast milk, and its use during breast-feeding is not known to be safe.

Class IV antiarrhythmic drugs

Verapamil has been used fairly commonly during pregnancy to treat cardiac arrhythmias, and there are no known adverse effects to the fetus. The drug does inhibit uterine contractions, which in fact has led to its use in inhibiting premature labor. Verapamil is excreted into breast milk but has no known adverse effects on nursing babies.

Diltiazem has been used much less frequently than verapamil during pregnancy. Little is known about its safety, though adverse effects have not been reported. It is excreted into breast milk and, ideally, should be avoided in mothers who are breast-feeding.

Nondrug antiarrhythmic therapy in pregnancy

Implantable defibrillators

The presence of an implantable cardioverter defibrillator (ICD) during pregnancy has not been associated with poor outcomes for either the mother or the fetus. Specifically, complications with ICDs do not appear to increase with pregnancy, nor do the frequency of ICD shocks.

Implanting an ICD during pregnancy is a much more difficult issue because of the necessity to use fluoroscopy. In general, pregnant women should not be exposed to radiation for any reason. If an ICD is deemed necessary for the mother's survival, the procedure can be considered—but the mother would need to be fully informed of the risks, and if an ICD is chosen, the procedure must be conducted with every precaution, including shielding of the mother (to the fullest extent possible) and the baby, and keeping the use of fluoroscopy to an absolute minimum.

Radiofrequency ablation

Radiofrequency ablation generally requires the use of large amounts of fluoroscopy, far more than would be required for implantation of an ICD, for instance. Therefore, this procedure should virtually never be performed during pregnancy—again, with the exception of a life-threatening arrhythmia for which no other viable treatment option exists.

Index

acid-base disturbances, 13, 26, 28*t*
acidosis, 47, 66
acute cardiac ischemia, 13
acute myocardial ischemia, 26, 75
adenosine, 108–109
  adverse effects, 109
  for AV node reentrant
    tachyarrhythmias, 108
  effect on tachyarrhythmias, 109*t*
α-adrenergic receptor blocking
    drugs, 43–44
adverse effects
  of adenosine, 109
  of amiodarone, 93–95
  of beta-blocking drugs, 84–85
  of calcium-blocking agents,
    105–106
  of Class I drugs, 76 (fig.)
  of disopyramide, 63
  of dofetilide, 100–101
  of flecainide, 74–75
  of ibutilide, 98
  of lidocaine, 67
  of mexiletine, 68
  of moricizine, 79
  of phenytoin, 70–71
  of procainamide, 61–62
  of propafenone, 77
  quinidine, 59–60
  of sotalol, 96–97
  of tedisamil, 116
adverse events, from
    antiarrhythmic drugs.
    See also proarrhythmias;
    torsades de pointes
  bradyarrhythmias, 95, 96, 109,
    117–118
  proarrhythmia, 116, 122–124

reentrant arrhythmia, worsening
    of, 118, 120–121
  worsening of hemodynamics, 122
afterpolarizations. *See* delayed
    depolarizations (DADs);
    early afterdepolarizations
    (EADs)
amiodarone, 40, 48, 87–95
  adverse effects/drug interactions,
    93–95
  clinical pharmacology, 90
  comparison with dronedarone,
    114–115
  dosage, 91–92
  electrophysiologic effects, 88, 90
  empiric therapy
    for hemodynamically unstable
      VT/VF, 160
    for sustained monomorphic VT,
      158
  indications, 92–93
  interactions
    digoxin, 108
    flecainide, 75
    procainamide, 61
  and proarrhythmia, 147
anorexia
  from amiodarone, 93
  from digoxin, 108
antiarrhythmic drugs. *See also*
    calcium-blocking agents;
    Class IA drugs; Class IB
    drugs; Class IC drugs;
    Class I: sodium-channel-
    blocking drugs; Class II:
    beta-blocking drugs; Class
    III drugs; Class IV drugs;
    individual drugs

antiarrhythmic drugs (*Cont.*)
aggressive *vs.* circumspect
approach, 133–134
and atrial flutter/atrial
fibrillation, 148*t*
avoidance of usage, 133
classification of, 42–51
Sicilian Gambit scheme, 49–51
Vaughan-Williams scheme,
43–49
effect on cardiac action potential,
36–38
effect on cardiac arrhythmias
automatic arrhythmias, 38
proarrhythmia, 40–42
reentrant arrhythmias, 40, 41
(fig.)
triggered activity
Brugada syndrome, 39–40
effect on ICDs, 128
effect on pacing thresholds, 128
mechanics of, 36–42
potassium blocking properties, 48
(fig.)
sodium blocking properties, 36,
43, 48 (fig.)
toxicity risks, 135*t*
anticholinergics
and disopyramide, 62, 63
interaction with quinidine, 60
and procainamide, 61
antihistamine agents, and ibutilide,
98
arthritis, from procainamide, 61
asthma, exacerbation of
from adenosine, 109
intravenous magnesium
treatment, 110
from sotalol, 96
ataxia
from amiodarone, 93
from mexiletine, 68
from phenytoin, 70
from propafenone, 77

atrial arrhythmias, 19, 26
and beta blockers, 82
and dronedarone, 115
drugs of choice for, 136*t*
treatment strategy, 20
Atrial Fibrillation Follow-up
Investigation of Rhythm
Management (AFFIRM)
trial, 144–145
atrial flutter/atrial fibrillation,
23–25, 140–150
consequences of
atrial kick loss, 141–143
tachycardia, 143
thromboembolism, 143–144
and dronedarone, 115
treatment of, 144–150
anticoagulation, 149–150
cardioconversion, 145–146
rate control, 146–147
rhythm control, 147–149
rhythm *vs.* rate control,
144–145
atrial tachyarrhythmias
and amiodarone, 92
and calcium-channel blockers,
104
and quinidine, 58
atrial tachycardia, 25, 104, 108,
118
atrioventricular (AV) groove, 3
atrioventricular (AV) node, 4, 24
(fig.), 49*t*, 80
sympathetic/parasympathetic
innervation, 10
atrioventricular nodal reentrant
tachycardias, 21–22
and adenosine, 107
and amiodarone, 92
and beta blockers, 81
and digoxin, 107
and quinidine, 58
automatic arrhythmias, 13, 19*t*, 28*t*,
38, 40

automatic atrial arrhythmias, 20,
    26
automatic atrial tachycardia, 12, 19,
    22, 24 (fig.)
automaticity, 4–5, 4 (fig.), 12–13
    abnormal
    and metabolic abnormalities,
        38
    in ventricular
        tachyarrhythmias, 26
    abnormal, in ventricular
        tachyarrhythmias, 26
    of AV node, 9
    suppression
        by beta-blockers, 80
        by calcium-blockers, 103
        by lidocaine, 66
        by quinidine, 57
automatic supraventricular
    tachyarrhythmias, 17–20
automatic tachyarrhythmias,
    12–13, 28t
    metabolic causes, 13
automatic ventricular
    tachyarrhythmias, 26
AV nodal reentrant tachycardia,
    21–22, 27t
    and adenosine, 108
    and calcium-channel blockers,
        104–105
azimilide, 112–114
Azimilide Postinfarct Survival
    Evaluation (ALIVE) trial,
    113

bepridil, 101
beta-blocking drugs. *See* Class II:
    beta-blocking drugs
binding kinetics drugs, 46 (fig.), 47
bradyarrhythmias, 95, 117–118
    from adenosine, 109
    from sotalol, 96
Brugada syndrome, 29, 33–34,
    39–40, 160

bundle branch reentry, 34t,
    161–162
bypass-tract-mediated
    macroreentrant
    tachycardia, 22, 74
bypass-tract-mediated tachycardias,
    58, 74, 78, 107, 164

calcium-blocking agents, 17. *See also*
    diltiazem; verapamil
    adverse effects/interactions,
        105–106
    clinical use
        atrial tachyarrhythmias, 104
        AV nodal
            reentry/macroreentrant
            tachycardias, 104–105
        multifocal atrial tachycardia,
            104
        supraventricular
            tachyarrhythmias,
            103–104
        ventricular tachyarrhythmias,
            105
    and DADs/EADs, 103
    electrophysiologic effects, 103
    suppression of automaticity, 103
cardiac action potential, 5–9, 5
    (fig.)
    depolarization phase, 6–7
    and EADs, 39
    effect of antiarrhythmic drugs,
        36–38
    relationship with surface ECG,
        10–12
    repolarization phase, 7–8
    resting phase, 8–19
Cardiac Arrest in
        Seattle-Conventional
        versus Amiodarone Drug
        Evaluation (CASCADE)
        trial, 158
Cardiac Arrhythmia Suppression
    Trial (CAST [1]), 74, 122

cardiac tachyarrhythmias
mechanisms
automaticity, 12–13
channelopathies, 16–17
reentry, 13–16, 14 (fig.), 15
(fig.)
triggered activity, 17
channelopathic ventricular
tachyarrhythmias,
28–34
Brugada syndrome, 33–34, 160
catechol-dependent triggered
arrhythmias, 29
pause-dependent triggered
arrhythmias, 29, 31–33, 33
(fig.)
triggered ventricle activity, 29
channelopathies, 16–17
chloramphenicol
interaction with mexiletine, 68
cimetidine
interactions
beta blockers, 85
dofetilide, 101
flecainide, 75
lidocaine, 67
mexiletine, 68
moricizine, 79
procainamide, 61
propafenone, 77
cinchonism, 59
cisapride, 101
Class IA drugs
causative for end-organ toxicity,
134
causative for torsades de pointes,
134
clinical pharmacology of, 57t
and defibrillation, 128
disopyramide, 44, 62–63
electrophysiologic effects of, 58t
exacerbation of reentrant
arrhythmias, 135
during pregnancy, 165

and proarrhythmias, 120
procainamide, 44, 60–62
quinidine, 44, 55–60
Class IB drugs, 63–71
and defibrillation, 128
lidocaine, 44, 64–67
mexiletine, 44, 67–68
phenytoin, 44, 69–71
during pregnancy, 165
tocainide, 44, 69
Class IC drugs, 71–79
and CAST, 122
and defibrillation, 128
electrophysiologic effects, 72t
encainide, 44, 75
exacerbation of reentrant
ventricular arrhythmias,
134
flecainide, 44, 72–75
moricizine, 44, 78–79
during pregnancy, 166
and proarrhythmias, 120
propafenone, 44, 75–77
Class I: sodium-channel-blocking
drugs, 37, 37 (fig.), 39–40
common adverse effects, 76 (fig.)
effects of binding kinetics, 46
(fig.), 47
inhibition of rapid sodium
channels, 36
Class II: beta-blocking drugs
adverse effects/drug interactions,
84–85
for arrhythmia treatment
supraventricular arrhythmias,
81–82
ventricular arrhythmias,
82–83
for atrial arrhythmias, 82
for AV nodal reentrant
tachycardias, 81, 82t
clinical pharmacology, 83–84
for congenital long QT-interval
syndrome, 82

electrophysiologic effects, 81
interactions
    amiodarone, 94
    sotalol, 96
for SA nodal reentrant
    tachycardia, 81, 82t
suppression of automaticity,
    80
Class III drugs
    amiodarone, 87–95
    azimilide, 112–114
    clinical pharmacology, 88t
    dofetilide, 98–101
    ibutilide, 97–98
    during pregnancy, 166
    sotalol, 95–97
Class IV drugs. See calcium-blocking
    agents
claudication, from beta blockers,
    85
clinical pharmacology
    of amiodarone, 90
    of beta-blocking drugs, 83–84
    of Class III drugs, 88t
    of diltiazem, 102
    of disopyramide, 62
    of dofetilide, 99
    of flecainide, 72
    of ibutilide, 97
    of lidocaine, 64–65
    of mexiletine, 68
    of moricizine, 78
    of phenytoin, 69
    of procainamide, 60
    of propafenone, 75
    of quinidine, 56
    of sotalol, 95
    of verapamil, 102
congenital long QT-interval
    syndrome, 82
congestive heart failure
    and disopyramide, 62, 63
    and flecainide, 74
    and ibutilide, 98

and moricizine, 78
and propafenone, 77
and quinidine, 56
and sotalol, 96
from sotalol, 96
and verapamil, 105
cyclosporine, 77, 105, 106, 111

DADs. See delayed depolarizations
    (DADs)
defibrillation, 128, 160. See also
    implantable cardioverter
    defibrillators (ICDs)
delayed depolarizations (DADs)
    from calcium-channel blockers,
        103
    from digoxin toxicity, 25, 121
    phenytoin suppression of, 70
    and polymorphic ventricular
        tachycardia, 121
    and repetitive monomorphic VT,
        162
    and triggered arrhythmias,
        39
depolarization phase, of action
    potential, 6–7
desipramine, 77
digoxin, 107–108
    adverse effects, 108
    for atrioventricular nodal
        reentrant tachycardias,
        107
    electrophysiologic effects, 107
    interactions
        amiodarone, 108
        erythromycin, 108
        flecainide, 75
        propafenone, 77
        quinidine, 60, 108
        tetracycline, 108
        verapamil, 108
diltiazem
    clinical pharmacology, 102
    dosage, 102–103

disopyramide, 44, 62–63
  adverse effects/drug interactions,
    63
  anticholinergic effects of, 62, 63
  clinical pharmacology, 62
  dosage, 62
  electrophysiologic effects, 62
  elimination/half-life, 62
  hemodynamic effects, 62
  interaction with phenytoin, 71
  oral administration, 62
  therapeutic uses, 63
dizziness
  from adenosine, 109
  from lidocaine, 67
  from moricizine, 79
  from propafenone, 77
  from quinidine, 59
  from verapamil, 105
dofetilide
  adverse effects/drug interactions,
    100–101
  clinical pharmacology, 99
  clinical use, 99–100
  electrophysiologic properties,
    98–99
  indications, 100
dosage recommendations
  for amiodarone, 91–92
  for diltiazem, 102–103
  for disopyramide, 62
  for flecainide, 72
  for ibutilide, 97
  for lidocaine, 65
  for mexiletine, 68–69
  for moricizine, 78
  for phenytoin, 69–70
  for of procainamide, 60
  for propafenone, 76
  for sotalol, 95–96
  for verapamil, 102–103
dronedarone
  for atrial fibrillation/atrial flutter,
    115
  Class I/IV properties, 114–115

drug-device interactions, 124,
  128–129
drug-drug interactions, 123,
  125t–127t
drug interactions
  of amiodarone, 93–95
  of beta-blocking drugs, 84–85
  of calcium-blocking agents,
    105–106
  of disopyramide, 63
  of dofetilide, 100–101
  of flecainide, 74–75
  of ibutilide, 98
  of lidocaine, 67
  of mexiletine, 68
  of moricizine, 79
  of phenytoin, 70–71
  of procainamide, 61–62
  of propafenone, 77
  of quinidine, 59–60
  of sotalol, 96–97
dry mouth, from disopyramide, 63,
  76t

early afterdepolarizations (EADs),
  31, 57
  and calcium-blocking agents
    potential, 103
  influence on cardiac action
    potential, 39
  and lidocaine, 66
  and pause-dependent ventricular
    tachyarrhythmias, 121
  and triggered arrhythmias, 39
electronic pacemakers, 118, 124
electrophysiologic effects
  of amiodarone, 88, 90
  of beta-blocking drugs, 81
  of calcium-blocking agents, 103
  of Class IA drugs, 58t
  of digoxin, 107
  of disopyramide, 62
  of flecainide, 73–74
  of lidocaine, 66
  of mexiletine, 68

of moricizine, 78
of phenytoin, 70
of procainamide, 61
of propafenone, 77
of quinidine, 56–57
electrophysiologic (EP) testing,
  156–157
electrophysiologic properties
of azimilide, 112
of cardiac tissue, 38
of Class IB drugs, 64
of Class III drugs, 89t
of dofetilide, 98–99
of flecainide, 74
of ibutilide, 97
of sotalol, 95
Electrophysiologic Testing versus
  Electrocardiographic
  Monitoring System
  (ESVEM) trial, 157
elimination/half-life
of adenosine, 108
of amiodarone, 90, 166
of digoxin, 107
of disopyramide, 62
of dofetilide, 99
of flecainide, 72
of ibutilide, 97
of lidocaine, 65
of mexiletine, 67
of moricizine, 78
of procainamide, 60
of quinidine, 56
of sotalol, 95
of verapamil, 102
empiric drug therapy
for hemodynamically unstable
  VT/VF, 160
for sustained monomorphic VT,
  158
encainide, 44, 75
clinical pharmacology (See
  flecainide)
electrophysiologic effects (See
  flecainide)

and sudden death, 122
epilepsy
from channelopathies, 17
EP testing. See electrophysiologic
  (EP) testing
erythromycin
interactions
digoxin, 108
dofetilide, 101
esophageal reflux
from amiodarone, 93
exanthematous pustulitis
from propafenone, 77

fever
from beta blockers, 85
from procainamide, 61
5-HT4 receptor antagonists. See
  piboserod
flecainide, 44, 72–75
adverse effects/drug interactions,
  74–75
binding kinetics, 46 (fig.)
and bypass-tract-mediated
  macroreentrant
  tachycardia, 74
clinical pharmacology, 72
dosage, 72
electrophysiologic effects, 73–74
elimination/half-life, 72
hemodynamic effects, 74
interactions
amiodarone, 94
and sudden death, 122
therapeutic uses, 74
flulike symptoms
from dofetilide, 100

gastrointestinal symptoms
from beta blockers, 85
from digoxin, 108
from dofetilide, 100
from flecainide, 74
from mexiletine, 68
from moricizine, 79

gastrointestinal symptoms (*Cont.*)
   from phenytoin, 70
   from quinidine, 59

half-life. *See* elimination/half-life
headaches
   from adenosine, 109
   from dofetilide, 100
   from moricizine, 79
   from quinidine, 59
heart, electrical system
   anatomy, 4 (fig.)
   cardiac action potential, 5–9
     depolarization phase, 6–7
     repolarization phase, 7–8
     resting phase, 8–19
   localized variations
     action potential differences,
      9–10
     autonomic innervation
      differences, 10
hemodynamically unstable VT/VF,
   160
hemodynamic effects
   of disopyramide, 62
   drug-induced worsening of, 122
   of flecainide, 74
   of lidocaine, 67
   of mexiletine, 68
   of moricizine, 78
   of phenytoin, 70
   of procainamide, 61
   of propafenone, 77
   of quinidine, 57–58
hemolytic anemia, 59, 76*t*
hepatic transaminases
   elevation
     from amiodarone, 93
     from verapamil, 105
hepatitis
   from amiodarone, 93
   from quinidine, 59
His-Purkinje system, 4, 5, 9, 10,
   105, 118

Holter monitoring, 147, 151,
   156–157, 158
hyperkalemia, 47
hyperthyroidism
   from amiodarone, 94, 166
   and atrial fibrillation/atrial
     flutter, 141*t*
hypoglycemia
   and beta blockers, 85, 166
   from disopyramide, 63
   and mexiletine, in newborn,
     165
hypokalemia, 13, 19
hypomagnesemia, 13, 19, 108, 111
hypoxemia, 13

ibutilide
   adverse effects/drug interactions,
     98
   clinical pharmacology, 97
   clinical utility, 98
   dosage, 97
   electrophysiologic properties, 97
   indications, 97
ICU arrhythmias, 13
idiopathic left ventricular
     tachycardia (ILVT), 34*t*,
     163
implantable cardioverter
     defibrillators (ICDs), 124,
     128
   effect of antiarrhythmic drugs,
     128
   for hemodynamically unstable
     VT/VF, 160
   during pregnancy, 167
   for sustained monomorphic VT,
     159
indications
   for amiodarone, 92–93
   for ibutilide, 97
   for sotalol, 96
interstitial fibrosis, chronic, from
     amiodarone, 93

investigational antiarrhythmic
    drugs
  azimilide, 112–114
  dronedarone, 114–115
  piboserod, 116
  tedisamil, 115–116
ischemia, 47
isoniazid, 68, 71, 125t, 126t

junctional tachycardia, 12, 108

lidocaine, 44, 46 (fig.), 64–67
  adverse effects/drug interactions,
    67
  binding kinetics, 46 (fig.)
  clinical pharmacology, 64–65
  dosage, 65
  electrophysiologic effects, 66
  hemodynamic effects, 67
  interaction with beta blockers, 85
  interaction with phenytoin, 71
  suppression of automaticity, 66
  therapeutic uses, 67
lupus
  from phenytoin, 70
  from procainamide, 60, 61
  from propafenone, 77
  from quinidine, 59

magnesium, 109–111
  and arrhythmias, 110
  oral/intravenous administration,
    111
  for supraventricular arrhythmias,
    110
  therapeutic uses, 111
  for torsades de pointes, 110
  toxicity symptoms, 110t
megaloblastic anemia, from
    phenytoin, 70, 76t
megestrol, 101
metoprolol, 67, 77, 83
mexiletine, 44, 67–68
  adverse effects, 68

clinical pharmacology, 68
dosage, 68–69
electrophysiologic effects, 68
hemodynamic effects, 68
interaction with phenytoin, 71
therapeutic effects, 68
migraine headaches, from
    channelopathies, 17
moricizine, 44, 78–79
  adverse effects/interactions, 79
  clinical pharmacology, 78
  dosage, 78
  electrophysiologic effects, 78
  hemodynamic effects, 78
  therapeutic uses, 78–79
multifocal atrial tachycardias
    (MATs), 13, 19, 20 (fig.),
    110
  and automatic atrial tachycardia,
    19
  and calcium-channel blockers,
    104
muscle disorders, from
    channelopathies, 17
myocardial function depression
  and beta blockers, 84
  and disopyramide, 63
  and quinidine, 58

nausea
  from amiodarone, 93
  from digoxin, 108
  from moricizine, 79
negative inotropy, from sotalol, 96
nonsustained ventricular
    arrhythmias, 151–155
nystagmus, from phenytoin, 70,
    76t

ocular symptoms
  from amiodarone, 94
  from digoxin, 108
osteomalacia, from phenytoin, 70,
    76t

pacemakers, electronic, 124
pacing thresholds, and
    antiarrhythmic drugs, 128*t*
paroxysmal atrial tachycardia,
    138–140
pause-dependent ventricular
    arrhythmias, 121
pause-dependent ventricular
    tachyarrhythmias, 121
pericarditis, 61
periodic paralysis, from
    channelopathies, 17
peripheral neuropathy, from
    amiodarone, 93
phenobarbital
    interactions
    disopyramide, 63
    lidocaine, 67
    propafenone, 77
    quinidine, 60
phenothiazines
    interactions
    dofetilide, 101
    ibutilide, 98
    quinidine, 60
phenytoin, 44, 69–71
    adverse effects/drug interactions,
        70–71
    clinical pharmacology, 69
    dosage, 69–70
    electrophysiologic effects, 70
    hemodynamic effects, 70
    interactions
    amiodarone, 94
    disopyramide, 63
    mexiletine, 68
    propafenone, 77
    quinidine, 60
    suppression of DADs, 70
    therapeutic uses, 70
photosensitivity, from amiodarone,
    93
piboserod (5-HT4 receptor
    antagonist), 116

pleuritis, from procainamide, 61
pneumonitis, from amiodarone, 93
polymorphic ventricular
    tachycardia, 121
potassium channel blocking drugs,
    44, 48 (fig.)
pregnancy
    drug treatment of arrhythmia
    Class IA drugs, 165
    Class IB drugs, 165
    Class IC drugs, 166
    Class III drugs, 166
    Class IV drugs, 167
    nondrug treatment of arrhythmia
    implantable defibrillators, 167
    radiofrequency ablation, 167
premature ventricular complexes,
    74
proarrhythmias, 117, 122–124
    and Class IA drugs, 120
    and Class IC drugs, 120
    drug-induced
    bradyarrhythmias, 117–118
    from flecainide, 75
    from moricizine, 79
    from propafenone, 77
    relative risk, 123*t*
    from tedisamil, 116
    torsades de pointes, 121
    worsening of hemodynamics,
        122
    worsening of reentry, 118,
        120–121
    effects of antiarrhythmicmic
        drugs, 40–42
    and sudden death, 120
    and torsades de pointes, 121
procainamide, 44, 60–62
    adverse effects/drug interactions,
        61–62
    anticholinergic effect, 661
    clinical pharmacology, 60
    dosage, 60
    electrophysiologic effects, 61

elimination/half-life, 60
hemodynamic effects, 61
interactions
  amiodarone, 94
oral/IV administration, 60
therapeutic uses, 61
prochlorperazine, 101
propafenone, 44, 75–77
adverse effects/drug interactions,
  77
clinical pharmacology, 75
dosage, 76
electrophysiologic effects, 77
hemodynamic effects, 77
therapeutic uses, 77
propranolol
interactions
  flecainide, 75
  lidocaine, 67
  propafenone, 77
proximal myopathy, from
  amiodarone, 93
pseudolymphoma, from phenytoin,
  70
pulmonary complications, from
  amiodarone, 93
Purkinje fibers. *See* His-Purkinje
  system

quinidine, 44, 55–60
adverse effects/drug interactions,
  59–60
for atrial tachyarrhythmias, 58
automaticity suppression in
  Purkinje fibers, 57
for AV nodal reentrant
  tachycardia, 58
for bypass-tract-mediated
  tachycardias, 58
clinical pharmacology, 56
electrophysiologic effects,
  56–57
elimination of, 56
hemodynamic effects, 57–58

interactions
  amiodarone, 94
  digoxin, 108
  propafenone, 77
interaction with flecainide, 75
interaction with phenytoin, 71
oral administration of, 56
sodium channel blocking effect,
  56–57
suppression of automaticity, 57
therapeutic uses, 58–59
vagolytic effect, 57–58
for ventricular tachyarrhythmias,
  58

radiofrequency ablation, 162, 163,
  167
rashes
from beta blockers, 85
from procainamide, 61
from propafenone, 77
from quinidine, 59
Rate Control *versus* Electrical
  Cardioversion (RACE)
  trial, 144–145
Raynaud's phenomenon, 84, 85
recurrent supraventricular
  tachyarrhythmias, 20–21
reentrant arrhythmias, 16, 28t, 119t
and adenosine, 108
effects of antiarrhythmicmic
  drugs, 40
exacerbation of
  by Class IA drugs, 135
  by Class IC drugs, 134
worsening of, 118, 120–121
reentrant atrial tachycardias, 81, 138
reentrant ventricular
  tachyarrhythmias, 26–28
reentry mechanism, cardiac
  tachyarrhythmia, 13–16,
  14 (fig.), 15 (fig.)
repetitive monomorphic VT
  (RMVT), 34t, 162

repolarization phase, of action
potential, 7–8
duration of, 11
phases of, 7
simultaneity of, 11–12
respiratory distress, from
amiodarone, 93
resting phase, of action potential,
8–19
rhythm/rate control, in atrial
fibrillation/atrial flutter,
144–145
rifampin
interactions
propafenone, 77
interaction with disopyramide,
63
interaction with quinidine,
60
right outflow tract tachycardia
(repetitive monomorphic
VT), 34t
right ventricular dysplasia, 161
RMVT. See repetitive monomorphic
VT (RMVT)

sexual dysfunction, from beta
blockers, 85
Sicilian Gambit classification
system, 49–51, 50 (fig.)
side effects. See adverse effects/drug
interactions
sinoatrial (SA) nodal reentrant
tachycardia, 81
sinoatrial (SA) node, 3
automaticity of, 118
dysfunction from digoxin,
108
sympathetic/parasympathetic
innervation, 10
sinus tachycardia, 12, 13, 25, 57
sleep disturbances
from amiodarone, 93
from dofetilide, 100

sodium channel blocking drugs, 36,
43, 48 (fig.), 56–57. See
Class I: sodium-channel
blocking drugs
sotalol
adverse effects/drug interactions,
96–97
clinical pharmacology, 95
dosage, 95–96
electrophysiologic properties, 95
indications, 96
sudden death
from Class IC drugs, 75
and encainide/flecainide, 122
patient risk categories, 151
and proarrhythmias, 120
from prolonged arrhythmic
episodes, 32
reduction of
from amiodarone, 92
from beta blockers, 82
risk from ventricular ectopy,
152t
supraventricular arrhythmias, 16
and azimilide, 113, 114
and beta-blocking drugs,
82–83
and magnesium, 110
supraventricular tachyarrhythmias
atrial flutter/atrial fibrillation,
23–25, 140–150
automatic supraventricular
tachyarrhythmias, 17–20
AV nodal reentrant tachycardia,
21–22
bypass-tract-mediated
macroreentrant
tachycardia, 22
and calcium-channel blockers,
104
ECG patterns, 26
intra-atrial reentry, 22
paroxysmal atrial tachycardia,
138–140

recurrent supraventricular
tachyarrhythmias, 20–21
SA nodal reentry, 25
triggered supraventricular
tachyarrhythmias, 25–26
surface electrocardiogram (ECG), 4,
10–12
sustained monomorphic VT. *See also*
repetitive monomorphic
VT (RMVT)
and Holter monitoring/EP testing,
156–157
treatment of, 155–159
acute treatment, 156
chronic treatment, 156–158
empiric drug therapy, 158–159
ICDs, 159
sustained ventricular arrhythmias.
See also nonsustained
ventricular arrhythmias
from ibutilide, 98
treatment of
hemodynamically unstable
VT/VF, 160
sustained monomorphic VT,
155–160

tachyarrhythmias
automatic tachyarrhythmias,
12–13
EAD-mediated tachyarrhythmias,
39
and magnesium, 109*t*
and reentry mechanisms, 13–16
relative efficacy for, 136*t*
tachyarrhythmias, clinical features
supraventricular
tachyarrhythmias
atrial flutter/atrial fibrillation,
23–25
automatic supraventricular
tachyarrhythmias, 17–20
AV nodal reentrant
tachycardia, 21–22

bypass-tract-mediated
macroreentrant
tachycardia, 22
ECP patterns, 26
intra-atrial reentry, 22
recurrent supraventricular
tachyarrhythmias, 20–21
SA nodal reentry, 25
triggered supraventricular
tachyarrhythmias, 25–26
ventricular tachyarrhythmias
automatic ventricular
tachyarrhythmias, 26
channelopathic ventricular
tachyarrhythmias, 28–34
miscellaneous ventricular
arrhythmias, 35
reentrant ventricular
tachyarrhythmias, 26–28
tachycardia zone, 16
tedisamil, 115–116
adverse effects, 116
Class III properties, 115
tetracyclic antidepressants, 31*t*,
98
tetracycline, 108
theophylline
interactions
moricizine, 79
propafenone, 77
interaction with phenytoin, 71
therapeutic uses
of disopyramide, 63
of flecainide, 74
of lidocaine, 67
of mexiletine, 68
of moricizine, 78–79
of phenytoin, 70
of procainamide, 61
of propafenone, 77
of quinidine, 58–59
thrombocytopenia
from mexiletine, 68
from quinidine, 59, 165

thyroid problems
from amiodarone, 93
from dronedarone, 114
tocainide, 44, 69
torsades de pointes, 17, 121
drug causations, 31*t*
antibiotics, 31*t*
class I/class II antiarrhythmic
drugs, 31*t*
phenothiazines, 31*t*
tricyclic/tetracyclic
antidepressants, 31*t*
from ibutilide, 98
and magnesium, 110
and proarrhythmias, 121
from sotalol, 96
from tedisamil, 116
toxicity risks, of antiarrhythmic
drugs, 135*t*
tremors, from amiodarone,
93
tricyclic antidepressants
interactions
dofetilide, 101
interaction with ibutilide,
98
triggered activity, 17, 37
and Brugada syndrome, 29,
160
effect of antiarrhythmic drugs,
39–40
pause-dependent, 32
and RMVT, 174
in ventricles, 29
triggered arrhythmias
caused by DADs, 39
caused by EADs, 39
triggered supraventricular
tachyarrhythmias, 25–26,
28*t*
trimethoprim
interactions
dofetilide, 101
procainamide, 61

unclassified antiarrhythmic agents
adenosine, 108–109
digoxin, 60, 75, 77, 107–108
magnesium, 109–111
urinary difficulties, from
disopyramide, 63

Vaughan-Williams classification
system. *See* Class IA drugs;
Class IB drugs; Class IC
drugs; Class I:
sodium-channel-blocking
drugs; Class II:
beta-blocking drugs; Class
III drugs; Class IV drugs
ventricular arrhythmias, 13, 16.
See also hemodynamically
unstable VT/VF; sustained
monomorphic VT;
sustained ventricular
arrhythmias
and beta-blocking drugs,
82–83
drugs of choice for, 136*t*
from ibutilide, 98
induced by quinidine, 59
pause-dependent, 121
significance of, 151–152
treatment of, 152–155
ventricular dysplasia, 34*t*
ventricular tachyarrhythmias
automatic ventricular
tachyarrhythmias, 26
and calcium-channel blockers,
105
channelopathic ventricular
tachyarrhythmias,
28–34
Holter monitor-
ing/electrophysiologic
testing for, 156
and lidocaine, 67
miscellaneous ventricular
arrhythmias, 35

and quinidine, 58
reentrant ventricular
    tachyarrhythmias, 26–28
and right ventricular dysplasia,
    161
uncommon, clinical features,
    34*t*
ventricular tachycardia
    from digoxin, 108
    polymorphic ventricular
        tachycardia, 121
ventricular tachycardia, w/right
    ventricular dysplasia,
    34*t*
verapamil
    interaction with dofetilide, 101

Veterans Administration Congestive
    Heart Failure
    Antiarrhythmic Trial
    (CHF-STAT), 153
vision, blurred
    from flecainide, 74
    from mexiletine, 68
vomiting
    from amiodarone, 93
    from digoxin, 108

warfarin
    interactions
        propafenone, 77
    interaction with amiodarone, 94
    interaction with quinidine, 60